INTRACELLULAR
PROTEIN
TURNOVER

ACADEMIC PRESS RAPID MANUSCRIPT REPRODUCTION

INTRACELLULAR PROTEIN TURNOVER

Edited by

Robert T. Schimke

Department of Biological Sciences
Stanford University
Stanford, California

Nobuhiko Katunuma

Department of Enzyme Chemistry
Tokushima University
Tokushima, Japan

Academic Press, Inc. New York San Francisco London 1975
A Subsidiary of Harcourt Brace Jovanovich, Publishers

ACADEMIC PRESS, INC.
111 Fifth Avenue, New York, New York 10003

United Kingdom Edition published by
ACADEMIC PRESS, INC. (LONDON) LTD.
24/28 Oval Road, London NW1

Library of Congress Cataloging in Publication Data

Symposium on Protein Turnover, Stanford University, 1973.
Intracellular protein turnover.

Bibliography: p.
Includes index.
1. Protein metabolism—Congresses. 2. Cell
metabolism—Congresses. 3. Cellular control mecha-
nisms—Congresses. I. Schimke, Robert T., ed.
II. Katunuma, Nobuhiko, (date) ed. III. Title.
QP551.S952 1973   574.1'33   75-1180
ISBN 0–12–625550–4

CONTENTS

v

221137

CONTENTS

CONTENTS

IV. SPECIFIC PROBLEMS IN TURNOVER OF PROTEINS

CONTRIBUTORS

Yoshiko Banno Department of Enzyme Chemistry, Institute for Enzyme Research, School of Medicine, Tokushima University, 3-Kuramoto-Cho, Tokushima 707

Diana S. Beattie Department of Biochemistry, Mt. Sinai School of Medicine, New York, New York 10029

Judith S. Bond Department of Biochemistry, Virginia Commonwealth University, Medical College of Virginia, Richmond, Virginia 23298

Matthews O. Bradley National Cancer Institute, National Institutes of Health, Bethesda, Maryland 20014

Ahmad Bukhari Biological Laboratories, Cold Spring Harbor Laboratory, Cold Spring Harbor, New York 11724

George W. Chang Department of Nutrition, University of California, Berkeley, California 94720

Kenji Chichibu Department of Enzyme Chemistry, Institute for Enzyme Research, School of Medicine, Tokushima University, 3-Kuramoto-Cho, Tokushima 707

Darrell Doyle Department of Molecular Biology, Roswell Park Memorial Institute, Buffalo, New York 14203

George A. Dunaway, Jr. Department of Biology, State University of New York, Buffalo, New York 14214

Edmond H. Fischer Department of Biochemistry, University of Washington, Seattle, Washington 98105

Paul J. Fritz Department of Pharmacology, Pennsylvania State University, College of Medicine, Hershey, Pennsylvania 17033

Alfred L. Goldberg Department of Physiology, Harvard Medical School, Boston, Massachusetts 02115

Yoshitaka Hamaguchi Department of Enzyme Chemistry, Institute for Enzyme Research, School of Medicine, Tokushima University, 3-Kuramoto-Cho, Tokushima 707

Norio Hayashi Department of Biochemistry, School of Medicine, Tohoku University, 2-1 Seiryo-Cho, Sendai 980

Helmut Holzer Biochemisches Institut, Universitat, Freiburg, Breisgau, Germany

Ronald W. Johnson Department of Pharmacology, New York University, School of Medicine, New York, New York 10016

Nobuhiko Katunuma Department of Enzyme Chemistry, Institute for Enzyme Research, School of Medicine, Tokushima University, 3-Kuramoto-Cho, Tokushima 707

Tsunehiko Katsunuma Department of Enzyme Chemistry, Institute for Enzyme Research, School of Medicine, Tokushima University, 3-Kuramoto-Cho, Tokushima 707

Francis T. Kenney Carcinogenesis Program, Biology Division, Oak Ridge National Laboratory, Oak Ridge, Tennessee 37830

Goro Kikuchi Department of Biochemistry, School of Medicine, Tohoku University, 2-1 Seiryo-Cho, Sendai 980

Haeng Ja Kim Department of Biochemistry, School of Medicine, Tohoku University 2-1 Seiryo-Cho, Sendai 980

Kaoru Kitajima Department of Medical Chemistry, Kyoto University Faculty of Medicine, Kyoto, Japan

Keiko Kobayashi Department of Enzyme Chemistry, Institute for Enzyme Research, School of Medicine, Tokushima University, 3-Kuramoto-Cho, Tokushima 707

Tatsuo Kokubu Department of Internal Medicine, School of Medicine, Osaka University, Fukushima-Ku, Osaka, Japan

Eiki Kominami Department of Enzyme Chemistry, Institute for Enzyme Research, School of Medicine, Tokushima University, 3-Kuramoto-Cho, Tokushima 707 Japan

Kai-Lin Lee Carcinogenesis Program, Biology Division, Oak Ridge National Laboratory, Oak Ridge, Tennessee 37830

Yoshiko Matsuda Department of Enzyme Chemistry, Institute for Enzyme Research, School of Medicine, Tokushima University, 3-Kuramoto-Cho, Tokushima 707

Takeo Matsuzawa Department of Biochemistry, School of Medicine, Fujita-Gakuen University, Toyoake 470-11, Japan

Glenn E. Mortimore Department of Physiology, Pennsylvania State University, School of Medicine, Hershey, Pennsylvania 17033

Shigetada Nakanishi Department of Medical Chemistry, Kyoto University Faculty of Medicine, Kyoto, Japan

Yasuo Natori Department of Nutritional Chemistry, Tokushima University, School of Medicine, Tokushima, Japan 707

Alice N. Neeley Department of Physiology, Pennsylvania State University, School of Medicine, Hershey, Pennsylvania 17033

Kazutaka Nishimura Department of Internal Medicine, School of Medicine, Osaka University, Fukushima-Ku, Osaka, Japan

Shosaku Numa Department of Medical Chemistry, Kyoto University, Faculty of Medicine, Kyoto, Japan

Akira Ohashi Department of Biochemistry, School of Medicine, Tohoku University, 2-1 Seiryo-Cho, Sendai 980, Japan

Kenneth Olden Department of Physiology, Harvard Medical School, Boston, Massachusetts 02115

Tsuneo Omura Department of Biology, Faculty of Science, Kyushu University, Kukuoka, Japan

Juraj Osterman Department of Pharmacology, Pennsylvania State University, College of Medicine, Hershey, Pennsylvania 17033

George M. Patton Department of Biochemistry, Mt. Sinai School of Medicine, New York, New York 10029

Martin J. Pine Department of Experimental Therapeutics and J. T. Grace Jr. Cancer Drug Center, Roswell Park Memorial Institution, Buffalo, New York 14203

Brian Poole Rockefeller University, New York, New York 10021

Walter F. Prouty Department of Physiology, Harvard Medical School, Boston, Massachusetts 02115

Kenneth M. Pruitt Laboratory of Molecular Biology, University of Alabama, Birmingham, Alabama 35233

Robert T. Schimke Department of Biological Sciences, Stanford University, Stanford, California 94305

Robert R. Schmidt Department of Biochemistry, Virginia Polytechnic Institute and State University, Blacksburg, Virginia 24061

Harold L. Segal Department of Biology, State University of New York, Buffalo, New York 14214

Taiichi Shiotani Department of Enzyme Chemistry, Institute for Enzyme Research, School of Medicine, Tokushima University, 3-Kuramoto-Cho, Tokushima 707

Hirobumi Tereaoko Department of Medical Chemistry, Kyoto University faculty of Medicine, Kyoto, Japan

John Tweto Department of Molecular Biology, Roswell Park Memorial Institute, Buffalo, New York 14203

Einosuke Ueda Department of Internal Medicine, School of Medicine, Osaka University, Fukushima-Ku, Osaka, Japan

Keiko Watarai Department of Biochemsitry, School of Medicine, Tohoku University, 2-1 Seiryo-Cho, Sendai 980, Japan

E. Lucile White Department of Pharmacology, Pennsylvania State University, College of Medicine, Hershey, Pennsylvania 17033

PREFACE

The Greek philosopher, Heracleitus, is the acknowledged exponent of the proposition that all "things" are in continual flux or change. This philosophical concept was translated into biological terms principally by Rudolf Schoenheimer some 2300 years later in the phrase "the dynamic state of body constituents." In the past 20 years there has been a growing interest in the processes and mechanisms whereby the cellular constituents of both uni- and multicellular organisms are replaced continuously. This interest has included not only the mechanisms and regulation of synthetic processes, but also the mechanisms and regulation of degradative processes. The increased awareness of the extensive and continual replacement of cellular proteins and its importance in determining developmental and adaptive phenomena in cells had led to the meeting of a group of 30 investigators to assess the available knowledge and to pose the unknowns of the properties and mechanisms whereby proteins are continually degraded.

This volume is the result of presentations of a Symposium on Protein Turnover held at Stanford University, Stanford, California on December 10-13, 1973, and included scientists from Japan and the United States. The papers cover a wide variety of areas related to protein turnover, including studies in bacterial systems, as well as cultured cells and intact animals, and deal with problems related to the properties of turnover, regulation of enzyme levels, as well as the physiological and enzymatic mechanisms whereby proteins are degraded.

The organizers of the Symposium express their appreciation to all the participants for the lively and informative exchange of information and ideas, to the Japan Society for the Promotion of Science and the National Science Foundation (United States) for its support, as well as that of Syntex Corporation of Palo Alto, and to Miss Marjorie Weessner and Mrs. Judith Lombardi for their excellent preparation of camera-ready copy of the manuscripts.

Protein Turnover in Microorganisms

DEGRADATION OF PROTEIN FRAGMENTS IN E. COLI

A. I. Bukhari

Cold Spring Harbor Laboratory
Cold Spring Harbor, New York 11724

Selective degradation of proteins is a well established but little understood biological phenomenon.
It is known that half-lives of proteins vary greatly
in eukaryotic cells. As discussed by Schimke (11) in
his review on the regulation of protein degradation
in mammalian tissues, some enzymes, such as tyrosine
transaminase, are turned over with half-lives as short
as 2 hours, whereas others persist in the cells for
days after synthesis. In the prokaryotic organism
Escherichia coli, preferential degradation of certain
polypeptides is very striking. Goldschmidt (5) demonstrated that prematurely terminated fragments of the
enzyme β-galactosidase disappear within minutes in
actively growing E. coli cells. The wild-type β-
galactosidase is completely stable under the same
conditions. These results were confirmed by Lin &
Zabin (7), who presented evidence that different
fragments of β-galactosidase are degraded at different rates. Specific proteolytic attack on a polypeptide was also shown for the L1 fragment of the
lactose (lac) operon repressor, which in contrast to
the repressor itself is highly susceptible to degradation (10). Similarly, the incorporation of various
amino acid analogues or puromycin into cell proteins
(4,9) and frequent errors in translation (4) lead to
rapid degradation of the resulting proteins. Apparently, E. coli has a protein degradation system which
can discriminate between normal and abnormal proteins.
The mechanism by which the aberrant polypeptides are
specifically degraded remains obscure.

3

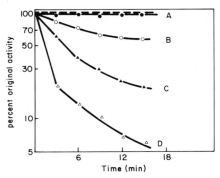

Figure 1: Degradation of β-galactosidase fragments in E. coli. Exponentially growing cells in standard LB broth at 37°C were induced with isopropyl-β-D-thiogalactopyranoside (IPTG, a gratuitous inducer of of the lac operon) at a final concentration of 5 x 10⁻⁴M. After 15-20 min growth in IPTG, cells were centrifuged, washed, and resuspended in warm broth and the incubation was continued on a shaker. The degradation of the β-galactosidase chains after removal of the inducer was followed by assay of auto-α donor activity. For details of the method, see Bukhari & Zipser (1973). The percent auto-α donor activity is plotted on a logarithmic scale as a function of time after removal of inducer.

(A) Wild-type β-galactosidase. Double line is meant to show that both auto-α activity and enzyme activity remain at the same level. (B) Auto-α of the X-90 fragment. (C) Auto-α of the 521 fragment. (D) Auto-α of the 545 fragment. The molecular weights of the X-90, 521, and 545 fragments, roughly estimated from the positions of these nonsense mutations in the lacZ gene (Fig. 2), are 120,000, 75,000, and 45,000, respectively (see also Morrison & Zipser, 1970).

A model system. The rapid degradation of the β-galactosidase fragments in E. coli provides a useful model for the study of selective protein degradation. The enzyme, which is a tetramer consisting of identical monomers of 135,000 mol. wt., is easy to assay (1). The monomer polypeptide can be conveniently resolved from other E. coli proteins by SDS-polyacrylamide gel electrophoresis (5,3). The gene coding β-galactosidase, the Z gene of the lac operon, has been dissected in great detail and the mechanics of its induction and expression are well understood (1). A wide variety of mutants producing amino-terminal or carboxy-terminal fragments of β-galactosidase, altered β-galactosidase monomers missing a few internal amino acids, complete but inactive β-galactosidase polypeptides, and conditionally active polypeptides have been isolated. The methods for assaying the mutant proteins are available. Thus, it is possible to induce a burst of synthesis of a mutant protein at any given time during the growth cycle of E. coli and to follow its intracellular fate accurately.

The assays for mutant β-galactosidase proteins are based on complementation between two enzymatically inactive polypeptides to give β-galactosidase activity (13). The complementation reaction occurs efficiently both in vivo and in vitro. A very useful in vitro assay is the auto-α assay, which specifically measures the amino-terminal part (the α region) of β-galactosidase (8). Auto-α is an amino-terminal peptide which is cleaved from a β-galactosidase chain upon autoclaving. It can complement the deletion 21 protein, which has a small deletion in the amino-terminal part of β-galactosidase, to give enzyme activity, and therefore the amount of auto-α can be estimated by mixing the autoclaved extract with the deletion 21 extract and measuring the β-galactosidase activity. We have exused the auto-α assay to study the kinetics of degradation of the amino-terminal part of the β-galactosidase mutant proteins in actively growing E. coli cells. The degradation of three β-galactosidase fragments of different sizes is shown in Fig. 1. Three

TABLE 1

In vivo complementation between Z nonsense mutations and
the amino-terminal Z deletions

Nonsense mutation	Deletion		
	Δ244	ΔB9	ΔR9
2579	-	-	-
2202	-	-	-
2540	-	-	-
2365	+	+	+
200	+	+	+
2444	+	+	+
X-90	+	+	+

The relative positions of the deletions (Δ) and the
nonsense mutations within the Z gene are given in Fig. 2.
The 244 and B9 deletion strains produce only the carboxyl-
terminal part of β-galactosidase. R9 is an internal
deletion, and thus in this case the middle part of the
enzyme is missing. All the nonsense mutants listed here
produce at least the amino-terminal part of the enzyme,
missing in the deletion strains. The nonsense mutations
are listed in order of the length of fragments they are
expected to produce. Thus, 2579 is closest to the operator
end of the gene and must produce the shortest fragment,
whereas X-90 is the farthest from the operator end and
therefore must produce the longest fragment among the mutations listed.

The complementation tests were done by mixing the F'
strains containing the Z deletions on F' lac episomes with
the F⁻ strains carrying the nonsense mutations, in drops on
Difco MacConkey and on minimal-lactose plates (Bukhari and
Zipser, 1972). Formation of Lac⁺ heterogenotes, and thus
generation of β-galactosidase activity by complementation,
was indicated by positive reaction on MacConkey (red color)
and growth on minimal-lactose plates. The + sign indicates
positive reaction within 10-24 hr. The - sign indicates no
reaction in 48 hr. It should be noted that the noncomple-
menting pairs here do complement when the deg mutants are
used, a result suggesting that the lack of complementation
is caused by degradation of the fragments.

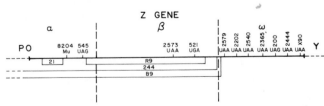

Figure 2: Genetic map of the lacZ gene. The α, β,
and ω regions of the Z gene are only approximately
defined by complementation. Terminating mutations
are shown above the line. Deletions are shown
below the line. The Symbol Mu indicates a terminating mutation caused by the insertion of phage Mu
DNA (Bukhari & Zipser, 1972).

6

points can be noted from the figure. First, the wild-
type β-galactisidase is completely stable, as indicated both by the native enzyme activity and by the
auto-α assay. Second, the auto-α activities of the
fragments decay rapidly, but they decay at different
rates. Third, the auto-α decay appears to be biphasic;
a fast decline in auto-α activity is apparently followed by a slower phase.

Rapid degradation of the β-galactosidase fragments
can be expected to interfere with the in vivo complementation reaction of these fragments. Complementation between some amino-terminal fragments, resulting
from the presence of nonsense mutations in the Z gene
and the carboxy-terminal fragments, produced because
of deletions of the amino-terminal part of the Z gene,
is shown in Table I. The location of the mutations
in the Z gene is given in Fig. 2. As can be seen in
the table, some pairs of mutations complement to give
β-galactosidase activity, and thus Lac⁺ cells, while
others do not. All of the nonsense mutations that
fail to complement a deletion are close to the end-
point of the deletion, an indication that the efficiency of complementation decreases as the length of
the overlap between the nonsense fragment and the
deletion fragment decreases. We have not observed
any case in which a long fragment clearly does not
complement a deletion but a shorter fragment does complement the same deletion fragment. Assuming that
the lack of complementation is primarily a consequence
of the degradation of the nonsense fragments, it can
be postulated that the degradation of the nonsense
fragments proceeds sequentially from the carboxyl-
terminal end. This is consistent with the observation
that the amino-terminal part of the large nonsense
fragments generally has longer half-life than the
amino-terminal part of the smaller fragments (Fig. 1).
The assumption that the inability of some pairs of
mutations to complement results at least in part from
the degradation of the nonsense fragments was proved
by the isolation of the E. coli mutants in which this
degradation is greatly reduced.

The degradation mutants. Bukhari & Zipser (2)
exploited the failure of complementation between some
pairs of lac mutations to isolate mutants of E. coli
that are defective in the degradation of the nonsense
fragments. The mutant selection strategy was to transfer an F' lac episome containing the ochre mutation
2540 in the Z gene to the mutagenized F⁻ recA⁻ (re-
combination-deficient) cells carrying the deletion
244 in the Z gene (Fig. 2), and to plate the mating
mixture on minimal medium plates with lactose as the
sole source of carbon. As shown in Table 1, 2540 and
Δ244 do not complement, and therefore the heterogenotes containing these two mutations do not have sufficient β-galactosidase activity to use lactose as
the carbon source. However, some Lac⁺ clones were
obtained from the 2540/Δ244 heterogenotes (approximate frequency being one Lac⁺ clone in 10^7 hetero-
genote cells), and these were found to be mutants in
which efficiency of 2540/Δ244 complementation had
been enhanced because of decreased degradation of the
2540 fragment. The degradation-defective mutants
have been termed the deg mutants. The effect of a
deg mutation on the large β-galactosidase fragment
X-90 is shown in Fig. 3. As reported originally by
Goldschmidt (5), the X-90 fragment rapidly disappears
in the wild-type E. coli cells. However, it is highly
stable in the deg⁻² mutants.

Characteristics of the deg mutants. The amounts
of all β-galactosidase fragments examined so far have
been found to increase in the deg mutants as compared
to the wild-type cells. Table 2 shows the effect of
deg mutations on the amino-terminal part of the β-
galactosidase fragments. Two points can be noted
from this table. One, all deg mutants have higher
amounts of auto-α than wild-type cells, but in none
of the mutants do the amounts of auto-α reach the
level expected if the degradation had completely
stopped. Thus, the deg mutations isolated are leaky;
the deg system continues to work, albeit at a slower
rate. Two, different deg mutants stabilize the same
fragment to different extents. This may simply reflect

8

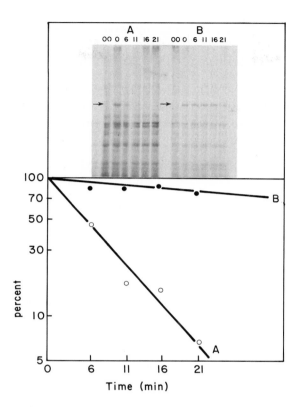

Figure 3: Decay of the intact X-90 fragment in the wild-type and the deg-2 mutant cells. The decay of the X-90 fragment was followed by pulse labeling of the fragment with ^{14}C-L-leucine and then examination of the fragment during the chase period by SDS-polyacrylamide gel electrophoresis. The experiment has been described in detail by Bukhari & Zipser (1973).

Upper half of the figure shows a part of the auto-radiograph. (A). Degradation of X-90 in the wild-type cells. (B). Degradation of X-90 in the deg-2 mutant. The position of the X-90 band is indicated by arrows. The time in minutes at which the sample was taken is indicated above each sample column. The first sample at left (00 sample) in both A and B is from cultures grown without IPTG, and therefore the X–90 fragment is not present. The relative densities of the X–90 bands at different times, obtained by scanning the film with a Joyce-Loebl microdensitometer, are plotted in the lower half of the figure. The amount of fragment just before chase (0-min sample) was called 100 and the percent radioactive fragment remaining was calculated accordingly.

TABLE 2

Effect of deg mutations on auto-α activity of the nonsense fragments of β-galactosidase

Fragment (Z nonsense mutations)	Strain	Auto-α (% wild-type β-galactosidase)
a. 2540	deg[+]	30
	deg-1	68
	deg-2	90
	deg-3	82
b. 521	deg[+]	6
	deg-1	32
	deg-2	73
	deg-3	51
c. 2573	deg[+]	1.5
	deg-1	6
	deg-2	8
	deg-3	6
d. 8204	deg[+]	0.2
	deg-2	4
e. 545	deg[+]	2.5
	deg-2	30
f. X-90	deg[+]	44
	deg-2	90

The Z nonsense mutations are shown in Fig. 2. Auto-α activity of a lac[+] wild-type strain was arbitrarily defined as 100, and other activities were normalized accordingly.

differences in the leakiness of mutations in the same
cistron, or it may mean that mutations are affecting
more than one gene controlling the deg system.

A comparison of the auto-α decay kinetics of the
521 and 545 fragments in the wild-type E. coli cells
(Fig. 1) and in the deg-2 mutant cells (Fig. 4) shows
that the deg mutation causes a four- to sixfold reduction in the rate of degradation of the amino-terminal
part of the fragments. The apparent biphasic nature
of the auto-α decay is absent in the deg mutant; instead, the auto-α decay follows a straight line. One
possible interpretation of this observation is that
the deg system is a multicomponent (or at least a two-
component) system and that the deg-2 mutation has
inactivated only one of the components.

The effect of the deg mutations on polypeptides
other than the β-galactosidase fragments has been
examined by Goldberg and coworkers (personal communication). They have found that the degradation of the
abnormal proteins that result from the incorporation
of puromycin is reduced two-fold in the deg mutants
as compared to the wild-type cells. Similarly, the
proteolysis that occurs in the E. coli cells after
the addition of amino acid analogs such as canavanine
is less extensive in the deg mutants. Apparently,
the mechanism by which the β-galactosidase fragments
are recognized as abnormal polypeptides is also involved in the recognition of other gross structural
defects in the protein molecules.

It was pointed out by Bukhari & Zipser (3) that
all the deg mutants isolated tend to be highly mucoid.
In the case of the deg-7 mutant, the mucoidy has been
shown to be the result of a mutation at the lon locus
(12). The mutations at the lon locus are known to
have pleiotropic effects in E. coli such as defect in
cell division, UV sensitivity, and derepression of
certain operons (6). It is possible that the deg
mutations are actually the lon mutations and that the
lon syndrome stems from an interference in the selective protein turnover in E. coli. However, it appears
more likely that the lon mutations in the deg mutants

11

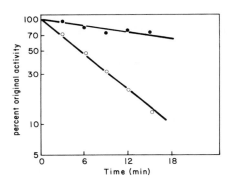

Figure 4: Degradation of the 521 and 545 fragments
in the deg-2 mutant cells. The degradation was
followed by the auto-α assay method as in Fig. 1.
Solid circles, auto-α decay of the 521 fragment in
the deg-2 mutant. Open circles, auto-α-decay of
the 545 fragment in the deg-2 mutant. See Fig. 1
for comparison of degradation of the same fragments
in the wild-type cells.

are merely superimposed on the unrelated deg mutations.
We have observed that spontaneously isolated lon mutants of the lacZΔ244 strain, originally used for the
isolation of the deg mutants, cannot complement the
appropriate nonsense mutations to give Lac+ clones.
Thus, by this criterion, none of the independently
isolated lon mutants have the deg phenotype. Furthermore, the strain used for the deg mutant selection
grows poorly on minimal medium at 37°C, but gives
fast-growing mutants at a high rate which always produce mucoid colonies. Since the deg mutants were
isolated at 37°C, it is likely that the lon mutations
were inadvertantly selected along with the deg mutations. The deg mutations are now being mapped accurately to resolve this point and to see whether they
fall in more than one gene.

The mechanism of degradation. The mode of degradation of the X-90 fragment has some interesting features. As reported by Goldschmidt (5), the intact
X-90 fragment completely disappears in the E. coli
cells. The half-life of the intact X-90 fragment
shown here in Fig. 3 is about 6 minutes. On the
other hand, the half-life of the X-90 auto-α, representing a polypeptide of about 7000 mol. wt. from the
amino-terminal end (8), is more than 30 min (Fig.1).
This is again consistent with the idea that the nonsense fragments are attacked sequentially from the
carboxy-terminal end. A carboxy-terminal specific
exopeptidase, for example, would first destroy the
integrity of the intact fragment, and would only later
reach the amino-terminal part of the fragment. However, the amount of auto-α from the X-90 fragment is
found to be quite high in the cells (44% of that expected from the wild-type β-galactosidase) despite
the fact that all of the intact fragment is susceptible to degradation. As was noted by Bukhari &
Zipser (3), this might mean that the deg system makes
cuts in the X-90 fragment, producing intermediates
which may not rapidly be digested into amino acids.
A possible model involving exoproteolytic and endo-
proteolytic attacks can be proposed to explain the

degradation of the X-90 and other nonsense fragments
of β-galactosidase. In this model, an exopeptidase
would first attack the fragment from the carboxy-terminal end. As the degradation proceeded, the conformation of the molecule would change, exposing sites
for the endopeptidase action. Some of the peptides
resulting from the endopeptidase cuts would be stable,
whereas others would be further digested into amino
acids.

It has been found that the carboxy-terminal fragments of β-galactosidase produced owing to the translation restarts within the Z gene are also degraded
rapidly in vivo (2). These restart fragments, which
are different from the nonsense fragments in that they
have the wild-type carboxyl end of the E. coli β-galactosidase, are not stabilized to any significant
extent in the deg mutants (B. N. Apte, unpublished
results). This is an intriguing observation since it
implies that at least some step involved in the degradation of the nonsense fragments is totally different
from that involved in the restart fragment degradation.
Potentially, another class of deg mutants, in which
the restart fragments are stabilized, can be isolated.
These mutants would help to throw light on the recognition mechanisms of the restart and nonsense fragments.

A characteristic feature of the deg system in E.
coli appears to be its energy dependence. As reported
by Goldberg (4) for protein breakdown in actively
growing cells, the in vivo degradation of the β-galactosidase fragments can be stopped by the energy-block-
ing agents. In the deg mutants the addition of potassium cyanide further stabilizes the fragments
(Shineberg, personal communication). Since normal
enzymatic reactions are not expected to be energy
dependent, this is consistent with the notion that
the deg system is a multiple-component system. The
energy-requiring step might be involved in making the
fragments available for degradation, and not in enzymatic degradation itself.

The studies on the degradation of proteins in E. coli have not provided any firm clues so far as to how the abnormal proteins are differentiated from the normal proteins. If the tertiary structure of a polypeptide determines its susceptibility to degradation, then some inactive but complete chains of β-galactosidase, having the wild-type amino-terminal and carboxy-terminal ends, should also be selectively degraded. We have recently isolated several mutants of E. coli in which lesions in the β-galactosidase protein make the enzyme either temperature sensitive or cold sensitive. In the temperature-sensitive mutants, β-galactosidase is active at 32°C but becomes inactive at 42°C. In the cold-sensitive mutants the enzyme is greatly activated at temperatures above 40°C. In one temperature-sensitive mutant, the β-galactosidase polypeptide remains stable at 42°C in the actively growing cells. Thus, in this particular case the gross change in structure does not makr the polypeptide for degradation. The degradation of the temperature-sensitive and cold-sensitive β-galactosidase proteins is being examined under different conditions to understand the relationship between the structure and polymerization of polypeptides and their susceptibility to degradation.

Acknowledgements

I wish to acknowledge support from the Jane Coffin Childs Memorial Fund for Medical Research (Grant #298). I am indebted to David Sipser for continuous encouragement and support.

References

1. Beckwith, J. R. & Zipser, D. (eds.). The Lactose Operon. Cold Spring Harbor Laboratory (1970).
2. Bukhari, A. I. & Zipser, D. Nature New Biol. 236, 240 (1972).
3. Bukhari, A. I. & Zipser, D. Nature New Biol. 243, 238 (1973).
4. Goldberg, A. Proc. Nat. Acad. Sci. U.S.A. 69, 422 (1972).

5. Goldschmidt, R. Nature New Biol. 238, 1151
    (1970).
6. Lieberman, M. M. & Markovitz, A. J. Bacteriol.
    101, 965 (1972).
7. Lin, S. & Zabin, I. J. Biol. Chem. 247, 2205
    (1972).
8. Morrison, S. L. & Zipser, D. J. Mol. Biol. 50,
    359 (1970).
9. Pine, M. J. Bacteriol. 93, 1527 (1967).
10. Platt, T., Miller, J. H. & Weber, K. Nature
    New Biol. 238, 1154 (1970).
11. Schimke, R. T. In Mammalian Protein Metabolism,
    Vol. IV, (H. N. Munro, ed), Academic Press,
    New York (1970).
12. Shineberg, B. & Zipser, D. J. Bacteriol. 116,
    1469 (1973).
13. Ullmann, A., Jacob, F. & Monod, J. J. Mol. Biol.
    24, 339 (1967).
14. Zabin, I. & Fowler, A. V. In The Lactose Operon.
    (J. Beckwith & D. Zipser, eds.) Cold Spring
    Harbor Laboratory (1970).

STUDIES OF THE MECHANISMS AND SELECTIVITY OF PROTEIN DEGRADATION IN E. Coli

Alfred L. Goldberg, Kenneth Olden,
and Walter F. Prouty

Department of Physiology
Harvard Medical School
Boston, Massachusetts 02115

Bacteria offer the biochemist enormous advantages for the study of metabolic processes, and in bacteria, as in animal cells, protein degradation appears to be a fundamental process whose mechanisms are still poorly understood (1-4). Nevertheless, until recently protein catabolism in bacteria was the subject of only limited study, probably because this process was widely believed to be of little physiological import. Such a conclusion is no longer tenable. It is now clear that E. coli, like mammalian cells, degrade a significant fraction of their proteins to amino acids even during exponential growth (5,6), that rates of proteolysis are carefully regulated, and change in response to variations in nutrient supply (1-8), and that different bacterial proteins turnover at nonuniform rates (5,6). The present article summarizes recent work in our laboratory on the control and mechanism of protein catabolism in E. coli and in particular on the selective degradation of abnormal proteins.

Regulation of Normal Protein Catabolism

It has been known for over twenty years that most proteins in E. coli are degraded relatively slowly during logarithmic growth but that this process increases two-to-four fold if cells are deprived of an

17

energy source, of nitrogen, or of a required amino acid (1-4). Recent studies by Dr. St. John in our laboratory have further shown that protein breakdown also increases when the cells are deprived of a variety of essential nutrients, including potassium, magnesium, sulfur, or phosphate (8)(St. John and Goldberg, in preparation). An acceleration of protein breakdown also occurs when most strains of E. coli enter stationary phase (Fig. 1). At the time when further growth ceases, degradation of cell protein increases dramatically. Resuspension of such cells in fresh medium leads to the reinitiation of growth and a rapid reduction in protein catabolism (Fig. 1). The increase in proteolysis during these various types of starvation of stationary phase does not reflect a loss of viability of the cells and does not occur when growth is simply prevented with inhibitors of RNA, DNA or protein synthesis.

Comparison of slowly growing and nongrowing cells further suggests that rates of protein catabolism are inversely related to cell growth (1, 9-12). The various conditions where protein degradation is augmented are also characterized by reduced synthesis of ribosomal and transfer RNA (Table 1), and there is now strong evidence that synthesis of stable RNA and protein degradation are regulated in a coordinated manner (1-3, 9-12). It has long been recognized that the production of ribosomes in E. coli is dependent upon the intracellular supply of aminoacyl tRNA (13). Various experiments from this laboratory have indicated that the supply of charged tRNA also influences the average rate of protein degradation (11). A typical experiment utilized mutants containing a temperature-sensitive valyl-tRNA synthetase. Such cells grown normally at their permissive temperature (30°), but cannot grow or form valyl-tRNA at 40°. When these cells are switched to 40°, rates of protein breakdown increased 9- to 12-fold even though they had a complete supply of amino acids. Similar findings were obtained in cells carrying temperature-sensitive

18

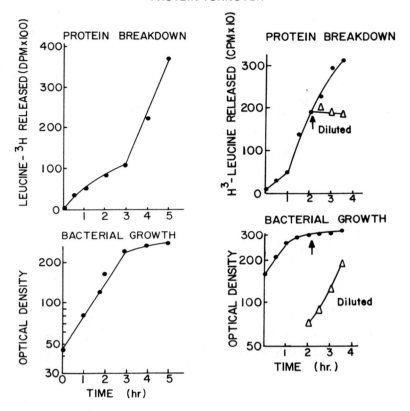

Figure 1. Protein Breakdown during Stationary Phase and Rapid Growth.

E. coli A33 grew exponentially for two generations on glucose-minimal medium supplemented with ³H-leucine. Figure 1A At zero time, the cells were deprived of the radioactive amino acid and were resuspended in growth containing large amounts of non-radioactive lecuine to prevent re-incorporation of radioactive amino acids released from protein. Degradation of protein was then measured as the release of ³H-leucine into acid-soluble form per ml of culture, as described previously (11). Figure 1B In a similar experiment, the cells in stationary phase were diluted 6 times in fresh medium and allowed to grow. The rate of protein breakdown after dilution was expressed as the rate per ml of undiluted culture. Growth was followed with Klett Summerson Colorimeter. No decrease in viability occured in cells at stationary phase.

TABLE 1

Factors Influencing Protein Degradation
and Ribosomal RNA Synthesis in E. Coli

	Protein Catabolism	RNA Synthesis
1) Stationary Phase	↑	↓
2) Starvation for		
a) Carbon Source	↑	↓
b) Required Amino Acids	↑	↓
c) Nitrogen	↑	↓
d) Potassium	↑	↓
e) Phosphate	↑	↓
f) Magnesium	↑	↓
g) Sulfur	↑	↓
3) Chloramphenicol in all types of starved cells	↓	↑
4) Blockage of formation of Valyl-tRNA	↑	↓
5) Trimethoprim or Hydroxyurea	↑	↓
6) Addition or Removal of cAMP	–	–

    The measurements of ribosomal RNA synthesis are based on published findings in many laboratories. Measurements of protein degradation are based on our own work and that of others (1-9). The enhancement of protein degradation generally ranged from 2-4 fold, although the observed responses varied in different strains. The inhibition of RNA synthesis was generally greater then 85%.

20

alanyl-tRNA synthetase and phenylalanyl-tRNA synthetase. When wild-type E. coli were switched from 30° to 40°, rates of protein degradation increased only 2- to 3-fold. Complementary experiments used various synthetic analogs of valine to block the synthesis of valyl-tRNA and trimethoprim or hydroxyurea to prevent formation of N-formyl methionyl-tRNA (11). Together these studies, which are analogous to earlier experiments on the control of RNA synthesis (13), indicated that the lack of a single charged species of tRNA leads to increased protein degradation at the same time that it inhibits synthesis of ribosomal RNA.

Previous work on the control of ribosome synthesis has concentrated on the relaxed (rel-) mutants (13), which fail to reduce RNA synthesis when they are deprived of a required amino acid or aminoacyl-tRNA. Experiments by Sussman and Gilvarg (10), our group (1,3), and Rafaelli-Eshkol and Hershko (14) have shown that most relaxed strains are also defective in their ability to regulate protein breakdown on amino acid starvation, although they give a relatively normal response with regard to RNA synthesis and protein degradation upon starvation for glucose and phosphate (1,10,14). Cashel and Gallant (15) have shown that normal (rel+) but not rel- strains accumulate high concentrations of guanosine tetraphosphate upon amino acid or nitrogen starvation. This nucleotide is synthesized by ribosomes of rel+ when they lack a single species of charged tRNA (16) or by all cells when they are starved for a carbon source (17,18). It is very attractive to hypothesize that this agent not only inhibits ribosomal RNA synthesis but also stimulates protein degradation.

The mechanism through which such an agent might alter the average rates of proteolysis is still unclear. It is noteworthy that protein degradation is maximally increased under certain conditions where protein synthesis is inhibited (Table 1). Thus it appears likely that increased degradation does not result from synthesis of new proteolytic enzymes but

instead from an activation of proteases that also
exist in growing cells. However, several groups have
found that chloramphenicol, an inhibitor of protein
synthesis, also retards the increase in protein
catabolism during starvation (1-4,14). This finding
was interpreted by some to indicate that starvation
leads to de novo synthesis of protelytic enzymes or
that protein degradation requires concomitant protein
synthesis (1-4, 14). However, chloramphenicol can
also lead to an accumulation of charged tRNA and can
directly reduce intracellular levels of guanosine
tetraphosphate (15, 18, 19). Thus the effect of inhibitors of synthesis on the degradative process is
probably an indirect one, as suggested previously (11).

These experiments thus also demonstrate interrela-
tionships between overall rates of protein synthesis
and degradation in the cell. Feedback mechanisms relating these two processes would seem highly advantageous to the organism. An adequate supply of charged
tRNA is obviously essential for ribosomal functioning.
When supply of these precursors is decreased, increased degradation of preexistent proteins would
serve to replenish amino acid pools and allow continued protein systhesis. In fact, in poor environments, protein catabolism appears to increase in
order that the cells can synthesize new enzymes
appropriate to the new conditions (1, 4, 20, 21). Unlike bacteria in adequate media, cells deprived of
essential amino acids or in diauxy lag (22) can obtain
necessary precursors for protein synthesis only from
preexisting cellular proteins. This argument predicts
that inhibition of protein degradation should also prevent new enzyme synthesis in starved cells but not in
growing cells (1, 20, 21). It is interesting in this
context that the various rel- strains have often been
selected because they adapt very slowly to "step down"
conditions and recover very slowly from stationary
phase. Such behavior can be explained by the failure
of rel- to increase protein catabolism under such conditions.

Such findings indicate that degradation of normal cell constituents serves an important adaptive function in "hard times". Consequently, it appeared possible that one stimulus for increased proteolysis was the accumulation of cyclic AMP in the starved cell. The increased levels of cyclic AMP at such times permit synthesis of messenger RNA for various catabolic enzymes (23). Some linkage between the control of protein degradation and catabolite repression appeared likely, since, as discussed above, increased proteolysis also appears essential for enzyme induction in starved cells (20, 21). Nevertheless, the addition of high concentration of cyclic AMP to growing or nongrowing cells did not augment protein breakdown, even though it did reverse catabolite repression in these cells. In addition, mutant strains (kindly provided by Dr. Ira Pastan and Dr. Jonathan Beckwith) that lack adenyl cyclase and can't synthesize cyclic AMP, still increased protein degradation upon starvation for glucose or amino acids. (Incidentally, the addition of cyclic GMP also did not appear to influence protein degradation.) Even though these experiments failed to demonstrate involvement of cyclic AMP in control of protein catabolism, changes in energy metabolism (e.g., upon glucose or phosphate deprivation) markedly influence rates of proteolysis. The mechanism of such effects are unknown, although supply of nutrients can cause accumulation of guanosine tetraphosphate by mechanisms apparently independent of the supply of charged tRNA (17, 18).

Catabolism of Abnormal Proteins in E. coli

In addition to its important function in the cell's adaptation to "hard times", protein degradation must serve an additional physiological role in growing cells (1, 24). There is now strong evidence that an additional important function of protein breakdown is the elimination of abnormal proteins from the cell (25, 26). Theoretically, such potentially harmful

polypeptides might be produced as a consequence of
mutation, mistakes in RNA or protein synthesis, chemical modifications of intracellular proteins, or even
"spontaneous" denaturation. Unfortunately, the frequency with which normal proteins denature within the
cell and the factors leading to irreversible denaturation are unknown. It is not unreasonable that all
enzymes within the cell might sooner or later be
subject to random chemical events leading to their
inactivation and unfolding (24). In any case, it is
likely   that strong selective pressures have caused
bacterial and animal cells to evolve degradative
mechanisms that insure that such aberrant, useless
polypeptides do not accumulate. The existence of
efficient degradative mechanisms in nongrowing cells
(e.g. mammalian cells) may in fact explain why the
protein composition of such cells can remain markedly
constant for long periods, even though the experience
of biochemists is that most protein structures are
highly labile at physiological temperatures.

Elegant genetic studies by Goldschmidt (27), Platt
et al. (28), Lin and Zabin (29), and Bukhari and Zipser
(30) on the lac operon have clearly documented that
E. coli can rapidly hydrolyze proteins resulting from
deletion or nonsense mutations. The normal products
of these genes are stable molecules, while the rapidly degraded proteins represent incomplete fragments
of β-galactosidase or polypeptides with altered
carboxyl terminal regions (the L-1 repressor). Additional evidence for the selective degradation of incomplete proteins comes from studies with puromycin
containing polypeptides (25, 26). Incorporation of
puromycin into a growing polypeptide leads to its pre-
mature release from the ribosome. The unfinished
polypeptides synthesized during exposure to low doses
of this agent are degraded much more rapidly than
normal cell constituents (Fig. 2)(25, 26). The
magnitude of this effect depends upon the amount of
puromycin present (Goldberg, unpublished observations)
and thus presumably on the percentage of incomplete

DEGRADATION OF PROTEINS CONTAINING

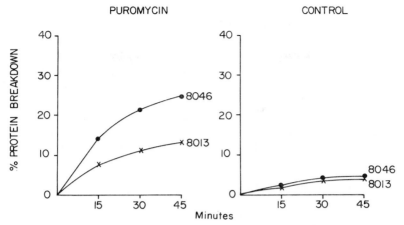

Figure 2. Fate of Puromycin-containing Polypeptides in Wild-type and deg-
E. coli.

Cultures of deg+ (8046) or deg- (8013) were incubated with or without
40 µg/ml of puromycin for 12 min. ³H-leucine was then added for five
minutes to label proteins. Both cultures were then filtered to remove ³H
and the drug. Protein degradation was then measured in the usual fashion
(11). Exposure to puromycin at this concentration inhibited incorporation
of ³H-leucine by 30%, but both cultures subsequently grew at the same rates.

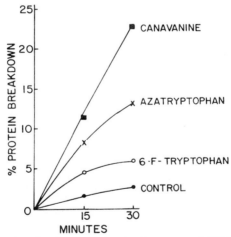

Figure 3. Fate of Proteins Synthesized in the Presence of Different Amino
Acid Analogs.

E.coli A33, an auxotroph for both arginine and tryptophan, was grown
initially in medium containing these amino acids. The cells were then
exposed for 5 min. to ³H-leucine in the presence of the required amino
acids or one of their analogs. Canavanine is incorporated in Protein in
place of arginine, and azatryptophan and 5-fluorotryptophan in place of
tryptophan. The labeled cells were then transferred to nonradioactive
medium containing the required amino acids, and the degradation of proteins
made in the presence of the analogs or the natural amino acids was measured
in the normal fashion. The rates of breakdown of labeled proteins are
expressed as the amount of ³H-leucine released into TCA-soluble form relative
to that initially present in the proteins. During the course of these measurements, the cells that had been exposed to the analogs grew at similar
rates as controls.

polypeptides synthesized. Puromycin only promotes
the degradation of proteins made in its presence;
since it does not affect preexistent polypeptides
within the same cell, these results are not a non-
specific effect of the antibiotic. Furthermore, experiments with ^{3}H-puromycin have shown it to be incorporated by growing bacteria into TCA-precipitable
material and then to be released as the puromycin-
containing polypeptides were selectively hydrolyzed
(25).

In addition, E. coli selectively degrade complete
poly-peptides, whose conformation is aberrant (25,26).
Large amounts of abnormal polypeptides are produced
when growing cells are exposed to various amino acid
analogs that are incorporated into proteins in place
of the normal residues. For example, auxotrophs requiring arginine can grow for several hours if supplied canavanine. However, the canavanine-containing
polypeptides are degraded from 4 to 10 times more
rapidly than those containing arginine (25). Experiments using acrylamide gel electrophoresis indicate
that the average size of proteins synthesized in the
presence of arginine and canavanine are not different
(Prouty and Goldberg, in preparation). In fact, the
molecular weights of a specific large polypeptide, the
monomer of β-galactosidase, are indistinguishable when
E. coli are induced in the presence of arginine or
canavanine (31). Under the latter conditions complete
but inactive β-galactosidase monomers are synthesized.
The analog-containing protein, unlike the normal
enzyme is then rapidly hydrolyzed, presumably as a
consequence of its abnormal conformation (31).

The hydrolysis of the analog-containing protein appears highly selective. In the same cell, proteins
containing trace amounts of ^{14}C-canavanine are degraded 3-5 times more rapidly than those containing [3]H-
arginine. Interestingly, the actual rate of degradation is dependent upon the extent of replacement of
the normal amino acids by the analog. For example,
incorporation of trace amounts of ^{14}C-canavanine in-

creased the absolute rate of proteolysis much less
than incorporation of large amounts of the analog.
Exposure of these cells to the large amounts of canavanine (1-20 μg/ml) can lead to extensive replacement
of the normal amino acid by the analog. Under these
conditions, protein conformations are probably affected to a greater extent than after incorporation of
trace amounts of the analog. Similarly, canavanine
had little or no effect on average protein half-lives
when given to wild-type cells, in which they fail to
compete effectively with the arginine that the cell
synthesizes.

Incorporation of a variety of other amino acid
analogs also promoted protein breadkown. Altogether,
14 different analogs were investigated, and all 14
were found to increase average rates of degradation
to some extent, although the magnitude of these
effects was quite variable. In general, those analogs
(e.g. fluorotyrosine or fluorotryptophan) that permitted relatively normal growth of the corresponding
auxotroph increased average rates of protein degradation less dramatically than canavanine (by about 50-
200%). By contrast, incorporation of certain other
analogs (e.g. azatryptophan, azetidine carboxylic acid,
canavanine) eventually blocks cell growth, and such
analogs promoted protein degradation dramatically
(from 4-10 fold). The varying effects of these different analogs presumably reflect the extent to which
the various analogs prevent the proteins from assuming
their normal tertiary conformations. In accord with
this view, those analogs that most effectively promoted protein degradation also prevented the formation
of enzymatically active β-galactosidase, while the
analogs that simulated degradation only slightly permitted the formation of apparently normal or temperature-sensitive enzymes (Goldberg, unpublished observations).

The finding that deviations from normal structures
markedly shorten protein half-lives _in vivo_ must mean
that normal proteins tend to share conformational

features distinguishing them from such rapidly degraded polypeptides. Unfortunately, these studies have not permitted a precise chemical definition of what the cell's degradative machinery recognizes as an abnormal protein. In this context, it is noteworthy that upon incorporation of a specific analog, average degradative rates obey complex, multi-component kinetics. These findings suggest that the incorporation of a specific analog can dramatically increase degradation of certain polypeptides, while the same analog has only mild effects on the turnover of other proteins. Presumably, such differences also result from the variable effects of a given analog on the conformation of individual cell proteins. Clearly, the use of amino acid analogs represents a useful experimental tool for the study of protein degradation, but the natural source of abnormal proteins (i.e. of substrates for this degradative system) is unclear. Possibly the rate-limiting step in the degradation of most cell proteins is their denaturation, leading eventually to their selective hydrolysis. Abnormal proteins may also arise as a consequence of mutations or mistakes in gene transcription and translation. In fact, protein degradation occurs several times more rapidly in bacterial strains that produce frequent errors in protein synthesis either because of a mutation in the ribosome (i.e. ribosomal ambiguity mutant, ram-) or in tRNA (supressor tRNA) (25) or because of treatment with streptomycin (26, 32). This difference in degradation probably reflects the selective removal of abnormal polypeptides resulting from synthetic errors, since revertant strains with normally accurate protein synthetic apparatus (ram+, su+) show normal rates of catabolism. The frequency of transcriptional and translational errors in normal cells is unknown. Previous attempts to determine such rates may have given inordinately low estimates because of the rapid elimination of the abnormal proteins.

Unlike normal proteins, whose degradation increases several fold upon starvation, the analog-containing

and puromycin-containing polypeptides are degraded
at similar rates in growing and starving cells (25).
Thus the catabolism of normal and aberrant proteins
appears to be regulated in distinct fashions possibly
through distinct mechanisms (21, 25). Two other experimental findings bear upon the latter conclusion:
1) Protease inhibitors which block the increase in
proteolysis in starved cells do not reduce the rapid
degradation of analog-containing proteins by growing
cells. These results are consistent with the existence of two proteolytic systems: one activated
during starvation and one present in all cells for
the hydrolysis of abnormal constituents. Unfortunately, the selectivity of such protease inhibitors has
been questioned (8), and their mechanism of action
in E. coli remains to be proven. 2) In addition,
Bukhari and Zipser have isolated mutants (deg-) defective in their ability to degrade nonsense fragments
of β-galactosidase. We have found that such strains
also degrade puromycin-peptides (Fig. 2) and proteins
containing azatryptophan (unpublished observations)
less rapidly than wild type. The deg- cells thus
appear to be defective in their ability to hydrolyze
aberrant proteins. However, the deg- cells also show
a slight reduction in the degradation of   normal
proteins during growth (Fig.2) and a slight reduction
in protein degradation during starvation (unpublished
observations). Thus if the bacteria do in fact contain two distinct degradative systems, they may well
share common elements.

The Energy Requirement for Proteolysis

One puzzling aspect of intracellular protein degradation is that this process appears to require metabolic energy (4, 25, 33-39). In E. coli (4, 25, 33) as
in slices of liver (35, 37), kidney(38), cultured
fibroblasts (35) or hepatoma cells(34), protein
catabolism can be inhibited by various procedures
that reduce the cell's capacity for glycosis or oxidative phosphorylation. It is intriguing that

metabolic inhibitors do not block protein turnover in disrupted preparations of liver; thus the apparent energy-dependence appears to require some degree of cellular integrity (37). The nature of this energy requirement is unclear since no known proteolytic enzyme of bacterial or mammalian origin requires ATP or other high-energy compounds. Furthermore, on thermodynamic grounds, this energy requirement is especially paradoxical, since the hydrolysis of peptide bonds should release energy.

Like the catabolism of normal bacterial proteins (1,4), the rapid degradation of proteins containing amino acid analogs or puromycin can be reduced by 70–90% by uncoupling agents, such as dinitrophenol or carbonyl cyanide-p-trifluoromethoxy-phenylhydrazone (25). Blockage of protein degradation in starved cells also occurs with azide or cyanide (25); these latter effects are reversible and thus can not be explained simply by cell injury or death (Fig. 4). Additional experiments have shown that this reduction in proteolysis is not a secondary effect of the blockage of protein synthesis that occurs when energy metabolism is inhibited (33).

Such findings suggest an obligatory coupling of metabolic energy to a step in protein catabolism. The inhibition of proteolysis has been generally attributed to a reduction in the steady-state level of ATP, but direct evidence for this conclusion was lacking. One important argument against this view is that ATP levels can be reduced to very low levels in E. coli (and in hepatocytes (34) or cultured fibroblasts (35)) without a reduction in proteolysis (Fig. 5) (33). In addition, other energy-linked functions in bacteria that have long been thought to be energized by hydrolysis of ATP (e.g. amino acid transport) can be driven by the cyclic oxidation and reduction of membrane proteins, which leads to the generation of a pH gradient or electrical potential across the cell membrane. Such an "energized membrane state" (40, 41) in turn may be the direct source of energy for many mem-

PROTEIN TURNOVER

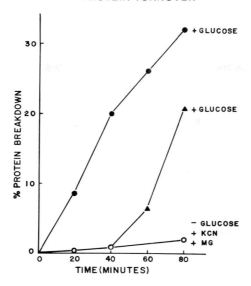

Figure 4. Energy Requirement for Degradation of Protein Containing Canavanine.

E. coli A33, an auxotroph for arginine, was grown to half saturation density, washed and exposed for 10 min. to ^{14}C-canavanine (0.05 μCi/ml) in arginine-free medium. The labeled cells were filtered and resuspended in medium containing 250μg/ml of arginine to prevent reutilization of ^{14}C-canavanine. For half the culture, protein degradation was measured in the presnece of glucose (i.e. in the growth medium); the other half was suspended in glucose-free medium containing potassium cyanide (1mM) and α-methyl-glucoside (20 MG, 20 mM). At 40 minutes, part of the latter culture was washed and resuspended in medium containing glucose.

At various times, 1.0 ml aliquots were taken and combined with TCA to make a 10% solution. Part of the TCA-supernatant was taken for determination of radioactivity. The amount of ATP in these aliquots was then assayed with the firefly luciferase assay as described by Stanley and Williams (51).

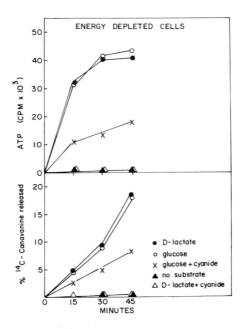

Figure 5. Recovery of Intracellular ATP and Protein Turnover in Energy-depleted E. Coli A33.

The cellular protein was labeled with ^{14}C-canavanine as described in Fig. 3. The cells were separated from the medium and washed thrice with ice-cold Tris (0.03 M, pH 7.0) medium. They were depleted of endogenous energy reserves by incubation in Tris medium containing α-methylglucoside (20 mM), arsenate (20 mM), and cyanide (1mM) for 90 min. at 37°. The cells were washed by filtrationand finally resuspended in phosphate-containing medium without metabolizable substrate (▲), or with D-lactate (0), D-lactate plus 1 mM cyanide (△), glucose (o), or glucose plus 1 mM cyanide (X).

brane-bound reactions.

Consequently, experiments were undertaken to define more critically how specific impairments in energy metabolism may affect protein degradation. These experiments generally followed the degradation of proteins containing ^{14}C-canavanine in an arginine auxotroph in the presence or absence of selective inhibitors. Initial experiments investigated the effects of cyanide, a potent inhibitor of cell respiration, in the presence or absence of glucose. If proteolysis is energized by electron transport, addition of cyanide should prevent protein hydrolysis. If protein catabolism is dependent upon substrate-level phosphorylation, cyanide should have no effect. In fact, protein breakdown was not inhibited when bacteria were incubated with KCN (1mM) in the presence of glucose (10mM) even though the level of ATP was reduced markedly (by 80-90%)(33). However, in the absence of glucose, cyanide inhibited proteolysis by about 70%, and ATP levels fell below 5% of control levels. These experiments thus indicate that glycolysis can provide sufficient energy for degradation of abnormal proteins.

Degradation of canavanine-containing proteins was inhibited almost completely (>95%) when α-methyl glucoside (α-MG) was added simultaneously with the cyanide in order to deplete further the cell's stores of high energy phosphates(Fig.4). Similar results were obtained upon complete restriction of cellular energy conservation by addition of arsenate, which blocks substrate-level phosphorylation, and cyanide to prevent respiration. Together these agents caused an almost complete inhibition of protein degradation (33). Since energy derived from glycolysis is sufficient to support protein catabolism and since ATP levels can be reduced markedly without affecting proteolysis, the requirement for phosphate bond energy must be relatively low.

These experiments do not indicate whether phosphate-bond energy is directly coupled to the proteolytic process or whether this effect is mediated via the energy-rich membrane state. In fact, it is known that ATP derived from glycolysis can give rise to the energized membrane state upon hydrolysis by the membrane-bound Ca-Mg ATPase. Evidence was obtained that high energy phosphates can directly support proteolysis by using a Ca-Mg-ATPase negative mutant (AN-120). This mutant cannot form the "energy-rich membrane state" by ATP hydrolysis in the presence of an inhibitor of respiration; nevertheless, degradation of canavanine-containing peptides occurred normally when this strain was incubated with cyanide and glucose (33).

E. coli contain sufficient stores of metabolizable substrates to meet their energy demands during starvation for several hours. Presumably these energy reserves allow the cell to degrade abnormal proteins even when deprived of an exogenous carbon source. In order to define more precisely the relationship between the rates of proteolysis and energy metabolism, the endogenous energy reserves were depleted by incubation in medium containing α-methyl glucoside, cyanide, and arsenate. (This procedure described in Fig. 5 was found to be highly effective and rapid, and far more convenient than other protocols for depletion of cell energy stores.) In such energy-depleted cells, protein degradation does not occur unless the cell is supplied exogenous substrates. Addition of glucose restored protein degradation whether or not cyanide was present. D-lactate, and oxidative substrate, permitted protein degradation but D-lactate was without effect if the cells were incubated with cyanide so as to block oxidative phosphorylation. However, neither glucose nor D-lactate were able to restore protein degradation if the cells were incubated with arsenate and thus unable to synthesize high energy phosphates. Under these conditions, respiration still occurred and was able to provide energy for active transport of proline. Thus, the capacity of these substrates to restore proteolysis correleates with their ability to generate high energy phosphates.

Such results also argue against the direct participation of glycolytic metabolites, such as PEP or hex-

ose phosphates, in the catabolic process. Unfortunately, these data do not provide information as to
whether the crucial energy source is ATP or another
nucleotide, or alternatively whether the accumulation
of monophosphate or diphosphate upon ATP-depletion
is inhibitory.

The nature of the energy-dependent reaction remains
an outstanding unsolved problem that is fundamental
to a complete understanding of the degradative process.
In eukaryotic cells, the energy-requirement for protein degradation has been generally explained by involvement of ATP in the function of the lysosome, the
presumed (but unproven)site of intracellular degradation. Conflicting evidence has been presented by
different groups for involvement of ATP in either
the maintenance of the pH gradient across the lysosomal membrane (42), or for transport of protein
into such structures (43, 44). In bacteria, the
energy-dependent step is even more uncertain (if
that is possible) because the site of the catabolic
process is unknown. Possible explanations of these
findings include an energy-dependent proteolytic
enzyme, or an energy requirement for the activation
of the responsible protease or for the modification
of protein susbtrates (e.g. analogous to the CoA-
derivatives of fatty acids). It is also possible
that the bacteria contain a degradative organelle
analogous to the lysosome that is still to be identified; for example, proteolytic enzymes exist in high-
est concentrations in the periplasmic fraction (Kowit
and Goldberg, unpublished observations), and energy
may be required to pump the abnormal protein into
that space. Despite appreciable effort, we have been
repeatedly unable to obtain definitive information
for any of these hypotheses.

Formation of Proteinaceous Inclusions During the Degradative Process

While attempting unsuccessfully to identify intermediates in the degradative process and to learn more

35

about the apparent energy-requirement, we made certain initially puzzling observations. When E. coli that had been exposed to canavanine for a short period were allowed to grow in the presence of arginine, they degraded 50% of the analog-containing proteins to TCA-soluble form during the subsequent hour (Fig. 3). Under these conditions, however, we were unable in repeated experiments to observe any loss of labeled, analog-containing proteins from the 100,000 g supernatant (45). This result was not anticipated because normally after sonication most of the proteins in E. coli are soluble upon centrifugation at 100,000 g. These findings indicated that the proteins selectively degraded by the cell must have been localized in some rapidly sedimenting centrifugal fraction (45). Further studies demonstrated that proteins synthesized in the presence of canavanine or various other amino acid analogs (31, 45) (Fig. 6) (Table 2) accumulate within granules sedimenting at 10,000 g. Normally, this fraction contains less than 5% of the cell proteins. However, the specific activity of canavanine containing proteins within the 10,000 g pellets was 25-40 times greater than in the supernatant, and 35-45% of the proteins synthesized in the presence of canavanine was recovered in this fraction (45).

Various observations suggest that the accumulation of analog-containing proteins in rapidly sedimenting particles is closely linked, perhaps even an essential step, in the degradative process. After removal of the analog, greater than 85% of the labeled protein in the 10,000 g was lost concomitant with the rapid protein degradation (Fig. 7, Table 2). In fact, loss of radioactivity from the particulate fraction could account for nearly all of the abnormal protein hydrolyzed to acid-soluble components. Analogous experiments with other amino acid analogs and puromycin (Table 2) also demonstrated a marked accumulation of the abnormal proteins in rapidly sedimenting fractions, and the magnitude of this effect correlated with the subsequent rate of protein degradation. Interestingly, when protein catabolism was prevented by blocking

TABLE 2

Relationship Between Size of 10,000xg Pellet and Subsequent Protein Breakdown

Proteins Synthesized in Presence of:	% Total Radioactive Protein in Cell		
	Degraded in 60 Min.	Initially in Pellet	Lost from Pellet in 60 Min.
EXP 1			
Arginine, Tryptophan	5	5.4	1.0
Arginine, 5-Fluorotryptophan	11	15	13
Arginine, Azatryptophan	23	20	14
Canavanine, Tryptophan	48	43	37
EXP 2			
Puromycin	50	26	22
EXP 3			
Lysine	5.8	7.0	0.4
β(Aminoethyl) cysteine	36	40	30

In Exp. 1, cells of E. coli A33, auxotrophic for both arginine and tryptophan, were collected during logarithmic growth, and resuspended in medium lacking the required amino acids. The culture was divided and the required amino amino acid or analog was added. The cultures were incubated for 12 min. and then [^{3}H]leucine was added to each flask for 5 min.

In Exp. 2, cells of 27873 growing in minimal medium received puromycin (100 μg/ml) for 12 min. prior to addition of [^{3}H]leucine for 5 min.

In Exp. 3, cells of 27798, a lysine auxotroph, were collected during logarithmic growth, and resuspended in glucose-minimal medium containing either lysine or S(β-aminoethyl) cystein. After 12 min., [^{3}H]leucine was added for 5 min.

After removal of [^{3}H]leucine and the analogs or puromycin, the cells were resuspended on the original growth medium supplemented with non-radioactive leucine. Protein degradation was measured as described previously (21) and expressed aʳ % of the radioactivity initially in protein that became acid-soluble. Aliquots were also taken for measurements of the amount of labeled protein sedimentable in 10 min. at 10,000g.

SUBCELLULAR DISTRIBUTION OF PROTEINS SYNTHESIZED IN PRESENCE OF

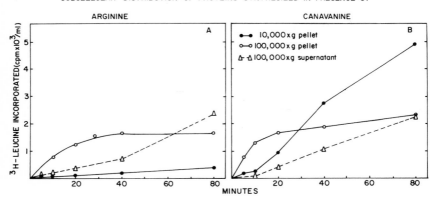

Figure 6. Subcellular Distribution of Newly Synthesized Protein During Growth on Arginine or Canavanine.

E. coli A33 were grown to late log phase on minimal medium containing arginine. At the start of the experiment, arginine and ^{3}H-leucine or canavanine and ^{14}C-leucine ware added to separate cultures. After addition of either compound, the doubling time of both cultures was 3.2 hours. At the times indicated, replicate 1.0 ml aliquots were removed and combined with carrier cells for measurement of radioactivity in the subcellular fractions of the sonicated cells, as described elsewhere. Total protein synthesis was determined by incorporation of radioactivity into TCA-precipitable material of whole cells, and in both instances appeared linear throughout the course of the experiment. Symbols are: X— X, 10,000g pellet; △——△, 100,000g pellet; and ◯---◯, TCA precipitate of 100,000g supernatant.

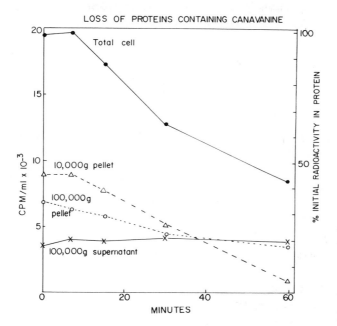

Figure 7. Loss of Proteins from Different Cell Fractions during Degradation of Canavanine-containing Proteins.

E. coli A33 during exponential growth was exposed to canavanine and ^{3}H-leucine as described in Table 3. Replicate 1.0 ml aliquots were removed at the times shown, combined with 4.0 ml carrier cells as described in Figure 6, and sonicated as described in Methods. Proteins in the 100,000 supernatant were precipitated with 5% TCA, and washed and counted as described previously (11). Loss of total cell proteins was measured as the decrease in TCA precipitable label in whole cells (45).

energy-metabolism, the loss of radioactive proteins from the pellets ceased, although labeled protein continued to accumulate within 10,000 g pellets.

These centrifugal pellets correspond to dense, a-morphous granules evident in cells exposed to canava-nine for even short periods (Fig. 8). The size and number of such osmiophilic granules increased with continued exposure to the analog (31). On the other hand, these inclusions disappeared upon resuspension of the cells in the presence of arginine. Under such conditions the particulate radioactivity was also lost as a consequence of the rapid degradation or the abnormal proteins. Similar structures have pre-viously been described by Schaetele and Rogers in cells killed after prolonged growth on high concen-trations of canavanine (46). These authors origin-ally suggested that the large inclusions of analog-containing proteins might be the cause of cell death. However, the cells studied here showed no decrease in growth rate or viability despite the presence of these large inclusions. Thus, the accumulation of abnormal proteins in granules and their subsequent hydrolysis may actually protect the cell from the harmful consequences of harboring abnormal proteins.

Because accumulation of proteins in these granules is closely linked to the degradative process, it appeared possible that these structures might repre-sent a degradative organelle analogous to the mammal-ian lysosome. However, electron micrographs and physichochemical studies suggested that they are not enclosed by a membrane (e.g. they are not sensitive to osmotic shock and are freely permeable to inulin) (31). Instead, they resemble dense aggregates of protein held together by noncovalent linkages. The analog-containing proteins within the 10,000 g pellets could be solubilized with sodium dodecyl sulfate but not with Triton X-100, dithiothreitol or NaCl. We have therefore solubilized the proteins accumulating in the 10,000 g pellets with sodium dodctyl sulfate in order to study their physical properties. Inter-

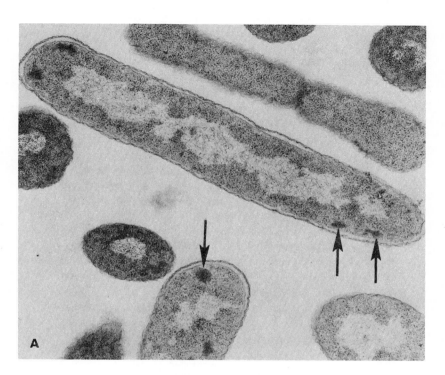

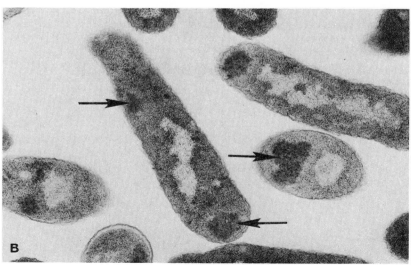

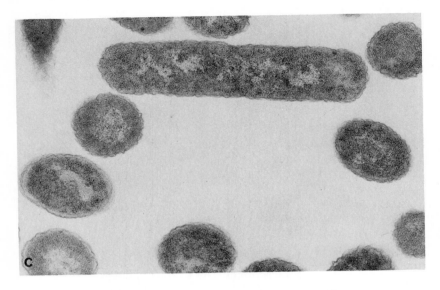

Figure 8. Electron Microscopy of Cells Exposed to Canavanine.

E. coli A33 were grown on glucose minimal medium to midlog phase. The cells were centrifuged, washed and resuspended in medium lacking arginine. Canavanine (20 μg/ml) was added to one portion and arginine to another. Aliquots from the culture containing canavanine were taken for microscopy after A) 15 minutes or B) 75 minutes. C) In addition, after 15 minutes exposure to canavanine, an aliquot was washed by filtration, and resuspended in the original growth medium containing arginine for one hour prior to electron microscopy. These aliquots were kept at 0° and then centrifuged at 5,000g for 10 minutes prior to fixation by an adaptation of the method of Kellenberger et al (52). Arrows indicate inclusions not found in control cells growing on arginine. The cells shown in C were indistinguishable from those in control cells never exposed to canavanine. All three are magnified 30,000 times.

estingly, if the ionic detergent is removed by dialysis, the canavanine containing proteins once again become rapidly sedimentable (31). Thus the proteins associated within the particulate fraction appear to be inherently less soluble than those in the 100,000 g supernatant, and it appears unnecessary to hypothesize the existence of a specific granule-forming process.

These observations and others suggest that the granules represent intracullular aggregates of denatured proteins, similar to those seen in various human diseases where large amounts of abnormal proteins are synthesized (e.g. thallasemia or Heinz-body anemia). Most likely the granules form spontaneously whenever cells produce large amounts of such insoluble components. Such granules are not demonstratable when cells are exposed to only trace amounts of ^{14}C-canavanine such that the amount of analog-containing protein per cell is low.

Electrophoretic studies of the isolated 10,000 g pellets have ruled out the possibility that the analogs cause the cell to synthesize specifically a class of insoluble (e.g. membrane-bound) proteins. Instead, the presence of analogs in polypeptides appears to alter their solubility properties. For example, after incorporation of canavanine, the normally soluble monomers of β-galactosidase are found associated with the 10,000 g pellets. It is interesting that after incorporation of the analogs, the larger polypeptides of the cell tend to be degraded especially rapidly, and such large polypeptides tend to be found disproportionately within the 10,000 g pellets (manuscript in preparation). This latter observation may be related to the findings of Schimke and coworkers (24, 47) that in general large polypeptides in eukaryotic cells tend to have shorter half-lives than smaller polypeptides (possibly the conformations of the larger polypeptides are more susceptible to denaturing influences).

Even though granule-formation and protein degradation appear to be closely linked, the present observations do not prove that the granules play an essential role in the degradative process. In fact, two
findings argue against such a conclusion: 1) Certain
mutations in the lac operon result in abnormal proteins that are soluble and rapidly hydrolyzed (27-30).
2) Upon incorporation of trace amounts of canavanine,
proteolysis is accelerated without a demonstrable increase in particulate radioactive protein. Even if
granule formation is not absolutely necessary for
rapid proteolysis, the spontaneous aggregation of the
abnormal proteins may serve to promote their recognition by the degradative system. Alternatively,
these inclusions may form only when the cell synthesizes abnormal proteins more rapidly than it can degrade them (e.g. upon incorporation of analogs or
puromycin). If the cell's degradative capacity is
saturated, the denatured proteins may then aggregate,
form inclusions, and remain in this state until the
degradative system can attack them.

Protein Half-Lives and Protease-Sensitivity

Perhaps the simplest biochemical model capable of
explaining the selective degradation of abnormal
proteins is that such polypeptides, because of their
conformations, are more susceptible to   digestion
by proteolytic enzymes than normal cell constituents
(48). Presumably normal cell proteins share conformational features that make them relatively resistant
to the cell's proteolytic machinery. It is likely
that deviations from such normal conformations--as
must occur in incomplete polypeptides, upon incorporation of amino acid analogs, or as a result of synthetic errors--would increase sensitivity to most
proteases. In fact, it has been known for over 30
years that once proteins are denatured, they are far
more susceptible to proteolytic hydrolysis (49).
(For this very reason, it is easier to digest a steak
that is first cooked, and probably for this reason,

our stomach produces an acid environment that is
effective in denaturing proteins.) In addition, this
simple generalization can account for the selective
degradation of abnormal proteins (48, 24).

Extensive experiments were pursued in this laboratory to test whether a general correlation might
exist between protein half-lives in vivo and their
sensitivity in vitro to various well-characterized
proteolytic enzymes. All experimental conditions
that promote the production of abnormal proteins
and thus increase the average rate of catabolism of
labeled proteins also increased their hydrolysis by
a variety of proteolytic enzymes (48), including
trypsin, chymotrypsin, papain, and pronase (Fig. 9).
In addition, we have found that specific mutant proteins that are rapidly degraded in E. coli, such as
the L-2 lac repressor, were also more sensitive to
proteolytic digestion in vitro than the wild-type
proteins (Table 3).

A variety of evidence further indicates that these
alterations in protease-sensitivity are responsible
for the enhanced rates of proteolysis in vivo. For
example, those analogs, whose incorporation most
markedly promoted intracellular proteolysis, also were
most effective in increasing susceptibility to pan-
creatic proteases. In addition, when E. coli that
had been exposed to canavanine were allowed to grow
in the presence of arginine and to degrade the analog-containing proteins, the susceptibility of the
cell extract to digestion by trypsin or papain decreased accordingly.

These findings strongly suggest that the cell's degradative machinery and the model proteases were re-
cognizing similar aspects of protein conformation.
Thus it appears unnecessary to hypothesize a new
type of intracellular proteolytic apparatus whose properties are far more sophisticated than those of known
proteases. A variety of unpublished experiments
support the view that these differences in protease-
sensitivity occur because the abnormal proteins are

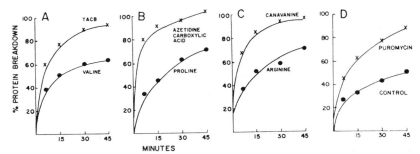

Figure 9. Comparison of Protease-sensitivity of Normal and Abnormal Proteins.

Correlation of protease-sensitivity and intracellular degradative rates: effect of trypsin (100 µg/ml) on proteins containing amino acid analogs or puromycin. Prior to lysis and incubation of cell extracts with trypsin, strain (A) M 48-62, a valine auxotroph, was exposed to ^{3}H-leucine and 50 µg/ml of either valine, or D,L-threo-α-amino-β-chlorobutyric acid (TACB), (B) M 55-25, a proline auxotroph, was exposed to ^{3}H-leucine and 20 µg/ml of either proline or azetidine carboxylic acid, (C) A33, an arginine and tryptophan auxotroph, was exposed to ^{3}H-leucine, tryptophan, and 20 µg/ml of either arginine or canavanine, (D) A33 was exposed to ^{3}H-leucine in the presence or absence of puromycin (300 µg/ml). Similar results were obtained with chymotrypsin, papain, and subtilisin.

EFFECTS OF TRYPSIN ON "STABLE" AND "RAPIDLY TURNING-OVER" E. COLI PROTEINS

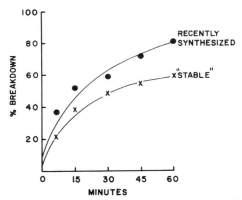

Figure 10. Comparison of Trypsin Sensitivity of E. coli Proteins with Different Intracellular Stabilities.

E. coli A33 was exposed to ^{3}H-leucine for 5 min. Half the culture was frozen (recently synthesized), and the other half ("stable") grew for two generations (2 hr) in the presence of nonradioactive leucine, during which time the cells degraded 8% of the labeled proteins to acid-soluble form. These cells, which had lost the more-labile cell proteins, were then frozen. Before preparation of the extracts and treatment with trypsin (100 µg/ml), the cells frozen initially were combined with nonradioactive cells to give comparable amounts of protein.

46

TABLE 3

COMPARISON OF PROTEASE-SENSITIVITY OF WILD-TYPE AND MUTANT REPRESSORS

Proteolytic Enzyme	Type of Repressor	^{14}C-IPTG Binding Activity		% Loss of Activity
		Initial Activity (cpm)	After Protease (cpm)	
Trypsin	wild-type	1970	1874	5
	L-1	508	263	48
Chymotrypsin	wild-type	1995	2155	0
	L-1	548	301	45
Subtilisin	wild-type	2032	2113	0
	L-1	398	255	36
Papain	wild-type	1960	1866	4
	L-1	458	279	39
None	wild-type	1960	1942	1
	L-1	538	544	0

The L-1 repressor is rapidly degraded in vivo, ($t_{1/2}$ <20 min), while the wild-type protein is stable. The wild-type and mutant (L-1) lac repressors were isolated according to the method of Platt et al (28) using strains M96 and 29-1. These strains carry a temperature-inducible defective prophage containing an i-promoter mutation (i^{SQ}) such that following induction the repressor constitutes nearly 2% of total cell proteins. Partially purified cell extracts were incubated at 37° with the protease at a final concentration of 91 μg/ml. Incubations were carried out for 30 minutes at which time loss of binding activity appeared maximal. In no instance was a significant effect on the wild-type observed. The amount of repressor was routinely assayed from the binding of ^{14}C-isopropyl-β-D-thiogalactoside (^{14}C-IPTG) by a modification of the assay of Bourgeois and Riggs (53). Following incubation with protease, 25 μl aliquots were removed and combined with 75 μl of buffer and 100 μl of ^{14}C-IPTG (2×10^{-6}M) at 4°. The samples were kept on ice for 10 minutes and then washed onto ice-cold Millipore filters with 2 ml. of cold buffer. These differences in protease-sensitivity were independent of the concentrations of the repressor molecules.

47

partially or completely denatured. For example, incubation of normal cell proteins in the presence of 1% sodium dodecyl sulfate or at 50° increased their sensitivity to trypsin and papain, until the arginine containing proteins were digested as rapidly as those containing canavanine. Similar treatment of canavanine-containing cell proteins did not further increase their digestion by these proteases (in preparation).

The correlation between protease-sensitivity in vitro and intracellular half-life can not only explain the selective catabolism of abnormal polypeptides, but also raises the possibility that differences in protease sensitivity might be responsible for the differences in the half-lives of normal proteins. To test this hypothesis (48), growing E. coli were administered a radioactive amino acid and either frozen immediately or allowed to grow for several generations and to degrade the labeled proteins. In the frozen cells, all types of proteins should be labeled. In the cells allowed to grow, polypeptides with shorter half-lives should have been selectively lost, and the proportion of labeled proteins with long half-lives should have increased. In fact, with time, susceptibility of cell proteins to trypsin decreased progressively. These studies thus indicated that the proteins most stable in vivo were also most resistant to trypsin and pronase (Fig. 10).

Incidentally, we have also obtained evidence for a correlation between intracellular degradation rates of proteins and protease-sensitivity with various eukaryotic cells, including cultured baby hamster kidney cells, rat liver, kidney, and brain (1,3). Extensive studies of a similar type have been carried out by Dice, Dehlinger, and Schimke (47) on soluble proteins from several rat tissues and for various subcellular fractions of rat liver. In addition, Bond (50) came to similar conclusions by comparing protease sensitivity of various liver enzymes. In all these systems it was found that the more labile cell proteins are more easily digested by proteases than more stable intracellular constituents. Presumably the structural features distinguishing the short-lived enzymes are similar to but more subtle than the structural differences distinguishing abnormal proteins from average cell constituents. The identification of the conformational factors that determine protease sensitivity obviously bears great import for understanding the control of enzyme concentrations.

Although differences in protease sensitivity can probably account for the selective hydrolysis of abnormal proteins and for the wide variations in protein half-lives normally occurring in bacterial and animal cells, it appears unlikely that such simple arguments can explain all the specificity in protein catabolism. In starving E. coli, for example, we have failed repeatedly to demonstrate a general increase in sensitivity of proteins to endoproteases, even though overall degradative rates increase several fold. Various studies discussed elsewhere instead suggests the activation of new proteolytic enzymes during starvation (20, 21). Thus, on one hand, the basal rate of degradation of an individual enzyme appears to be determined by its inherent sensitivity to cell proteases (that is, by its tertiary conformation). On the other hand, physiological factors, such as supply of nutrients to the cells, alter overall degradative rates presumably by influencing the cell's proteolytic machinery or altering the protease sensitivity of cell proteins (24).

It is also obvious that simple differences in protease-sensitivity do not provide a precise mechanism for protein degradation and can not explain the two features of the degradative process discussed above: 1) the energy requirement, and 2) the accumulation of abnormal proteins in granules prior to their rapid hydrolysis. A major goal of future work will be to determine how these different findings can be related to one another in a coherent explanation of the degradative process.

SUMMARY

Although the overall rate of protein degradation is low in growing E. coli, this process increases several fold when the bacteria enter stationery phase or when they are deprived of required nutrients. Enhanced protein breakdown appears to be an important adaptation to poor environments and occurs simultaneously with reduced synthesis of ribosomal RNA. Various experiments suggest that protein breakdown is controlled by similar mechansims to those regulating biosynthesis of stable RNA.

Another important function of intracellular protein degradation is the selective removal of proteins having abnormal conformations. Both growing and non-growing cells rapidly hydrolyze incomplete polypeptides (e.g. puromycin-peptides) or complete proteins that have incorporated amino acid analogs or contain synthetic errors. Incorporation of different amino acid analogs have variable effects on degradative rate, and these differences probably depend on the extent to which they perturb normal protein conformations.

The degradation of analog-containing proteins is an energy-requiring process although cellular ATP can be significantly reduced before this process is inhibited. Substrate phosphorylation in glycolysis can provide sufficient energy for protein degradation. Experiments with selective inhibitors and energy-depleted cells indicate that intermediates in glycolysis or the "energized-membrane state" do not directly provide energy for protein degradation.

When large amounts of aberrant proteins are produced, they accumulate in rapidly-sedimenting granules prior to their hydrolysis. These granules correspond to dense osmiophilic inclusions evident

within such cells by electron microscopy. The intracellular inclusions are not membrane-bound, but appear to be amorphous complexes of the abnormal proteins. The loss of labeled proteins from such structures can account for nearly all of the protein being
degraded to acid-soluble material. These granules
probably form spontaneously by intracellular precipitation of the abnormal proteins. Unlike granule formation, the loss of proteins from these granules is
energy dependent.

The various types of abnormal proteins that are
selectively degraded by the bacteria (e.g. error containing proteins or the mutant lac repressor) are
also more sensitive to degradation in vitro by various
well-defined endoproteases. The enhanced protease-
sensitivity reflects the partially denatured character
of the analog-containing proteins. In addition,
those normal proteins that turn over rapidly during
exponential growth appear more sensitive to proteolytic digestion by these enzymes than more stable cellular components. Although a general correlation has
been demonstrated between in vivo stability of cell
proteins and their in vitro sensitivity to protelytic
enzymes, this principle can not explain the enhanced
protein-breakdown during starvation.

Acknowledgements

This work has been made possible by research grants
from the National Institute of Neurological Disease
and Stroke, the Muscular Dystrophy Association of
America, and Air Force Office of Scientific Research.

Alfred L. Goldberg holds a Research Career Develop-
ment Award from the National Institute of Neurological
Disease and Stroke. During most of this work, Dr.
Walter Prouty held a Postdoctoral Fellowship from
National Institute of Mental Health, Dr. Kenneth Olden

was supported by a grant from the Macy Foundation.

We are grateful for Dr. Ann St. John and Mrs. Elsa Fox for their assistance in the preparation of this manuscript.

References

1. Goldberg, A.L., Howell, E.M., Li, J.B., Martel, S. B. and Prouty, W.F. Fed. Proc. 33:1112-1120 (1974).

2. Pine, M.J. Ann. Rev. Microbiol. 26:103-126 (1972).

3. Goldberg, A.L. in Intracellular Protein Catabolism, symposium of the Biochemical Society of the DDR, 1974 (in press).

4. Mandelstam, J. Bacteriol. Rev. 24:289-308 (1960).

5. Nath, K. and Koch, A.L. J. Biol. Chem. 246:6956-6957 (1971).

6. Pine, M.J. Biochim. Biophys. Acta 104:439-456 (1965).

7. Ben-Hamida, F. and Schlessinger, D. Biochim. Biophys. Acta 119:183-191 (1966).

8. Schechter, Y., Rafaeli-Eshkol, D. and Hershko, A. Biochem. Biophys. Res. Commun. 54:1518-1524.

9. Pine, M.J. J. Bacteriol. 115:107-116 (1973).

10. Sussman, A.J. and Gilvarg, C. J. Biol. Chem. 244:6304-6306 (1969).

11. Goldberg, A.L. Proc. Nat. Acad. Sci. 68:362-366 (1971).

12. Pine, M.J. J. Bacteriol. 116:1253-1257 (1973).

13. Edlin, G. and Broda, P. Bacteriol. Rev. 32:206-226 (1968).

14. Rafaeli-Eshkol,D. and Hershko, A. Cell 2:31-35 (1974).

15. Cashel, M. J. Biol. Chem. 224:31-33 (1969).

16. Hazeltine, W., Block, R., Gilbert, W., and Weber, K. Nature 238:381-384 (1972).

17. Lazzarini, R.A., Cashel, M. and Gallant, J. J. Biol. Chem. 246:4381-4385 (1971).

18. Gallant, J., Margason, G. and Finch, B. J. Biol. Chem. 247:6055-6058 (1972).

19. Glazier, K. and Schlessinger, D. J. Bacteriol. 117:1195-1200 (1974).

20. Goldberg, A.L. Nature New Biol. 234:51-52 (1971).

21. Prouty, W.F. and Goldberg, A.L. J. Biol. Chem. 247:3341-3352 (1972).

22. Willetts, N.S. Biochem. Biophys. Res. Commun. 20:692-696 (1965).

23. Perlman, R.L. and Pastan, I. Current Topics in Cellular Regulation, N.Y. Academic Press, 1971, 117-134.

24. Goldberg, A.L. and Dice, J.F., Jr., Ann Rev. Biochem. (1974, in press).

25. Goldberg, A.L. Proc. Nat. Acad. Sci. 69:422-426 (1972).

26. Pine, M.J. J. Bacteriol. 93:1527-1533 (1967).

27. Goldschmidt, R. Nature 228:1151-1154 (1970).

28. Platt, T., Miller, J. and Weber, J. Nature 228: 1154-1156 (1970).

29. Lin, S. and Zabin, I. J. Biol. Chem. 247:2205-2211 (1973).

30. Bukhari, A.I. and Zipser, D. Nature New Biol. 243:238-241 (1973).

31. Prouty, W.P., Karnovsky, J.J. and Goldberg, A.L. J. Biol. Chem. (1974, in press).

32. Pinkett, M.O., Brownstein, B.L. J. Bacteriol (in press, 1974).

33. Olden, K. and Goldberg, A.L. Submitted for publication.

34. Hershko, A. and Tomkins, G.M. J. Biol. Chem. 246: 710-714 (1971).

35. Poole, B. and Wibo, M. J. Biol. Chem. 248:6221-6226 (1973).

36. Simpson, M.V. J. Biol. Chem. 201:143-154 (1953).

37. Brostram, C.O. and Jeffay, H.J. J. Biol. Chem. 245:4001-4008 (1970).

38. Steinberg,D. and Vaughan, M. Arch. Biochem. Biophys. 65:93-105 (1956).

39. Goldspink, D. and Goldberg, A.L. Biochem. J. 134: 829-832 (1973).

40. Klein, W.L. and Bayer, P.D. J. Biol. Chem. 247: 7257-7265 (1972).

41. Berger, E.A. Proc. Nat. Acad. Sci. 70:1514-1518 (1973).

42. Mego, J.L., Farb, R.M. and Barnes, J. J. Biochem. 128:763-769 (1972).

43. Huisman, W., Bouma, J.M.W. and Gruber, M. Nature 250:428-429 (1974).

44. Hayashi, M., Hiroi, Y. and Natori, Y. Nature New Biol. 242:163-166 (1973).

45. Prouty, W.F. and Goldberg, A.L. Nature New Biol. 240:147-150 (1972).

46. Schachtele, C.F. and Rogers, P. J. Mol. Biol. 33:843-860 (1968).

47. Dice, J.F., Dehlinger, P.J., and Schimke, R.T. J. Biol. Chem. 248:4220-4228 (1973).

48. Goldberg, A.L. Proc. Nat. Acad. Sci. 69:2640-2644 (1972).

49. Rupley, J.A. In Methods in Enzymology XI, 905-917 (1967).

50. Bond, J.S. Biochem. Biophys. Res. Commun. 43:333-339 (1971).

51. Stanley, P.E. and Williams, S.G. Anal. Biochem. 29: 381-392 (1969).

52. Kellenberger, E., Pyter, A. and Sechaud, J. J. Biophys. Biochem. Cytol. 4:671-678 (1958).

53. Riggs, A. and Bourgeois, S. J. Mol. Biol. 34:361-364 (1968).

THE REGULATION OF PROTEIN DEGRADATION IN THE BACTERIUM Salmonella typhimurium

George W. Chang

Department of Nutritional Sciences
University of California
Berkeley, California 94720

As Bukhari and Goldberg have already indicated (1, 5), there are many advantages in using bacteria for the study of protein turnover. Because of their rapid growth, simple nutrient requirements, and the ease with which their physiology and genetics may be manipulated, bacteria have been used very successfully for the investigation of basic biological processes such as protein synthesis, cell division, the regulation of gene expression, and the nature of the genetic code.

Bacteria also support protein turnover, and we hope that by studying the process in the bacterial system, we can help to construct a detailed and verifiable model for protein turnover in mammalian systems. Finally, as one of our nutritional science students pointed out, protein turnover seems to be especially important when bacteria are starved for nitrogen or carbon sources; in other words, we are studying protein-calorie malnutrition in bacteria!

In this paper I will present three aspects of our work with the bacterium Salmonella typhimurium, which is a close relative of the ubiquitous E. coli: (1) our method of measuring protein turnover, (2) our procedure for isolating protein turnover mutants, and (3) protein turnover levels in mutants with well-known biochemical lesions.

Measurement of Protein Turnover. Before we could
study protein turnover, we had to obtain reliable
methodology in our own lab. Of the various methods
reported, the decarboxylation method of Pine (7) seemed
to be the most convenient. In this method, E. coli
cells first incorporate 1-[^{14}C] leucine into protein.
Then they are washed and suspended in a high concentration of non-radioactive leucine, which equilibrates
rapidly with the intracellular leucine and prevents
the reutilization of the radioactive leucine released
in the course of protein turnover. Most, if not all,
of the radioactive leucine released in the course of
protein turnover accumulates in the medium. The radioactivity of the free leucine is measured conveniently
by decarboxylating the amino acid with ninhydrin and
measuring radioactive CO_2 released. Since only free
leucine is subject to decarboxylation, there is little
interference from leucine-containing peptides, and no
need to filter or centrifuge the radioactive suspensions.

Karen Fenton and I modified Pine's procedure in the
following ways (2): (1) When we harvest and wash the
bacteria, we use Nucleopore[R] filters, instead of
Millipore[R], Gelman[R], or Schleicher and Schuell[R] membrane filters. The Nucleopore filters do not have
the open mesh micro-structure which the other filters
have, and the recovery of free cells is much better.
The other membrane filters trap the cells very well,
but when we try to resuspend the cells, many of them
remain attached to the filter.

(2) Instead of decarboxylating the free amino acids
with ninhydrin, we use chloramine T. Chloramine T
decarboxylates amino acids more rapidly than ninhydrin
(8). The decarboxylation reaction is complete in minutes instead of hours.

The modified protein turnover assay is fast, convenient, and precise. We can handle dozens of samples
in about a half hour. Variation between replicate
samples is usually less than 5%. Our simplified procedure is especially suitable for routine work, even
though it lacks some of the refinements of Pine's
procedure.

Isolation of Protein Turnover Mutants. When studying any metabolic system in bacteria, it is usually
helpful to obtain mutants lacking that system. Biochemical and nutritional analyses of the mutants often
enable one to understand the cellular machinery involved.
In our case we wanted to isolate mutant bacteria which
had lost either their protein turnover machinery or
their ability to regulate protein turnover. These
mutants would have unusual patterns of protein turnover.

In order to select protein turnover mutants from a
randomly mutated population of cells, we had to guess
what the physiological behavior of a protein turnover
mutant would be. Then we had to devise an experimental
procedure which would allow us to isolate any bacteria
with that physiological behavior. Many workers in the
field have suggested that protein turnover is most
critical to starving cells. The amino acids released
can be utilized for the synthesis of new protein or
as a source of energy. If this is the case, a mutant
bacterium which could not support protein turnover
could probably not be induced to synthesize new enzymes
under starvation conditions. We looked for mutant bacteria which could not be induced to synthesize beta-
galactosidase under starvation conditions.

Craig Eldred, Dennis Federico, and I developed the
following procedure for isolating mutants:

1. Induce mutations in a suitable parent strain of
Salmonella typhimurium. The parent strains we use
have a number of convenient genetic characters including a proline requirement. Since they are Salmonella
strains, they cannot produce beta-galactosidase.

2. Introduce an unmutated beta-galactosidase gene
on an E. coli F'lac episome. The resulting bacterium
has a mutated Salmonella chromosome and an unmutated
set of E. coli genes coding for the enzyme we want to
induce, beta-galactosidase.

3. Plate out a few hundred cells on a petri dish
and allow colonies to develop. In practice, we com-
bine steps 2 and 3 by spreading a large excess of a
suitable F'lac donor strain on proline-deficient medium

and then adding a few hundred mutated recipient cells. The F'lac episome also carries proline genes, and only those mutated cells which receive an episome can form colonies.

4. Make a filter paper replica of the colonies on the plate. We press a sterile filter paper to the plate and then pull it off gently. Whenever there was a colony on the plate, there was a dab of that colony adhering to the paper. Since the filter paper contains very little nutrient, those dabs of bacteria on the paper are starving.

5. Incubate the filter paper with IPTG, an inducer of beta-galactosidase synthesis.

6. Assay the colonies on the filter paper for beta-galactosidase activity. This is done simply by adding a buffer solution containing 6-bromo-α-naphthyl-β-D-galactoside and the diazonium salt Fast Blue 2B. Those colonies which have synthesized beta-galactosidase turn purple, while those which have not synthesized the enzyme stay yellow.

7. By comparing the stained filter paper with the original plate (step 4), we can pick up part of those colonies corresponding to any interesting spots of stain. These are our potential protein turnover mutants.

We screened about 16,000 colonies and isolated 5 strains with the expected characteristics. Three of these strains grow very poorly on carbon sources such as glycerol, ribose, arabinose, and citrate. The strain with the lowest protein turnover and the least growth on citrate was TC132.

Characterization of Protein Turnover Mutant TC132. By inducing a homogeneous suspension of exponentially growing cells in liquid medium and then using a quantitative assay, we confirmed the inability of TC132 to support the induced synthesis of beta-galactosidase. For wild-type cells induced under growth conditions for one hour, we usually obtained specific activities of around 100 (μmoles per min per mg cells), and during starvation, the specific activity is 2-4. For mutant TC132 induced under growth conditions, the

specific activity is 95, and during starvation, less
than 0.2.

The protein turnover behavior of mutant strain
TC132 is shown in Table I. TC132 has an abnormally
low protein turnover rate during carbon starvation,
but essentially normal rates during growth and during
nitrogen starvation. Perhaps the strain has a regulatory defect which prevents it from increasing protein
turnover levels in response to carbon starvation.

At first glance, TC132 looks something like a mutant with a lesion in its cyclic AMP metabolism.
Adenylate cyclase (cya) mutants and cyclic AMP recep-
tor protein (crp) mutants cannot utilize a number of
poor carbon sources (6). Neither can TC132. Cya and
crp mutants have abnormal responses to carbon starvation.

Nevertheless, we do not think TC132 is a cyclic AMP
mutant: 1) Unlike cya mutants, TC132 does not respond
to exogenous cyclic AMP. This chemical has no effect
on the carbon utilization or protein turnover patterns
of TC132. 2) In preliminary genetic mapping experiments, Dennis Federico has tentatively located the
TC132 lesion close to the met E gene, at about 11
o'clock on the coli-Salmonella genetic map. This is
far from the crp locus. Reversion and transduction
experiments indicate that the poor carbon source utilization and the abnormal protein turnover pattern of
TC132 are due to a single genetic lesion. 3) Neither
cya nor crp mutants have abnormal protein turnover
patterns. Both are very similar to wild-type bacteria
under conditions of growth, carbon starvation, and
nitrogen starvation.

Protein Turnover in Mutants with Well-Known Bio-
Chemical Lesions. By using mutants with well-known
biochemical lesions, we can test some of the current
hypotheses about the regulation of protein turnover.
A possible involvement of aminoacylated tRNA was
reviewed this morning by Dr. Goldberg and will no
doubt be mentioned by Dr. Pine. If aminoacylated
tRNA's are involved in the regulation of protein
turnover, mutants producing abnormal tRNA's may show

TABLE I.

Protein Turnover Rates of Wild-Type Salmonella LT-2 and Strain TC132

Strain	Growth	C-starvation	N-starvation	N,C-starvation
	(glucose NH_4)	(NH_4)	(glucose)	(no additions)
LT-2 and other parental strains	2-3	6	5-6	5-6
TC132	3	3	6	8

Protein turnover (% per hour), under the above conditions (parentheses indicate the additions to the mineral base we use for our medium).

TABLE II.

Protein Turnover Rates (% per hour) in Nitrogen-starved Salmonella Mutants with Functional and Non-functional hisT Gene Products

HisT Function	Genotype	Genetic Background[1]	
		(A) No Suppressor	(B) Suppressor 500
YES	Wild-type (TA265	4.4	
	sup 500		5.0
	HisT2890 sup 500		4.9
NO	HisT2890	3.4	
	HisT1529	3.0	
	HisT1529 sup 500		3.5

[1] Columns A and B show the results for two isogenic series of bacteria. Strains TA265, hisT2890, and hisT1529 are genetically identical, except for their hisT alleles. Similarly, all the suppressor-carrying strains are identical, except for their hisT alleles. Since the genetic background influences the protein turnover levels, comparisons can safely be made within a given column, but comparisons between values in column A and those in column B are less reliable.

abnormal protein turnover patterns. Dr. Bruce Ames
in the Biochemistry Department at Berkeley has isolated several mutants which make abnormal tRNAs or
reduced levels of tRNA^{His}. These mutants were originally selected because they produced constitutively
high levels of the histidine biosynthetic enzymes. We
obtained several mutants from him and measured their
protein turnover levels under nitrogen starvation.

One class of histidine regulatory mutants, the hisT
mutants, lack one of the tRNA modification enzymes (4).
These mutants produce a set of tRNA's which are not
fully pseudouridylated and which do not function properly in the regulation of the biosynthesis of several
amino acids. If tRNAs are involved in the elevation
of protein turnover rates in response to nitrogen
starvation and if the undermodified tRNAs of the hisT
mutants will not function properly in the regulation
of protein turnover rates, then we would expect to
see abnormal turnover levels in hisT mutants. This
is exactly what is shown in Table II.

In Table II all the strains listed above the dotted
line have a functioning hisT enzyme. All of them have
elevated protein turnover levels under nitrogen starvation. All the strains below the dotted line lack the
hisT enzyme and have low levels of protein turnover.
There are a few controls included. HisT2890 has a UAG
(amber) termination codon in the interior of the cistron and produces a short, incomplete polypeptide produce (3). The incomplete polypeptide has no hisT enzymatic activity and the strain has a low turnover
rate. If the his T2890 allele is introduced into a
strain carrying a suitable UAG-suppressor locus (in
this case, suppressor 500), a complete hisT polypeptide is made, despite the UAG codon. Functioning hisT
enzyme is made and the bacterium can support high levels
of protein turnover, as the strain his T2890 sup 500
does. Finally his T1529 is not suppressed by sup 500.
Regardless of whether the his T1529 allele is in a
wild-type genetic background or a sup 500 background,
there is no hisT function and there are low turnover
levels.

63

The protein turnover levels observed in the various hisT mutants are consistent with the generally accepted idea that protein turnover levels are normally low, but can be elevated during starvation for carbon or nitrogen, and that tRNA's are involved in raising the turnover rate during nitrogen starvation. The fact that hisT mutants lack the specific pseudouridine modifications in the anticodon regions of several tRNA species suggests that the anticodon regions may be involved in the regulation of protein turnover.

References

1. Bukhari, A., these proceedings.
2. Chang, G. W. & Fenton, K. Analyt. Biochem., in press.
3. Chang, G. W., Roth, J. R. & Ames, B. N. J. Bacteriol 108: 410 (1971).
4. Cortese, R., Kammen, H. O., Spengler, S. & Ames, B. N. J. Biol. Chem. 4: 1103 (1974).
5. Goldberg, A. L., these proceedings.
6. Perlman, R. L. & Pastan, I. Science 169: 339 (1970).
7. Pine, M. J. J. Bacteriol. 115: 107 (1973).
8. Van Slyke, D. D., Dillon, R. T., MacFadyen, D. A. & Hamilton, P. J. Biol. Chem. 141: 627 (1941).

CONTROL OF INTRACELLULAR PROTEOLYSIS DURING
ENERGY RESTRICTION IN INTACT AND
PERMEABILIZED ESCHERICHIA COLI

Martin J. Pine

Department of Experimental Therapeutics
and J. T. Grace Jr. Cancer Drug Center
Roswell Park Memorial Institute
Buffalo, New York

Summary

Various modes of energy restriction have been examined for their effects on intracellular proteolysis in
E. coli. The energy supply has two opposing roles in
intracellular proteolysis, as a negative regulator and
an essential requirement. Thus, removal of glucose or
O_2, or inhibition of oxidative phosphorylation with
2,4-dinitrophenol or of fermentation with fluoride
individually stimulate but in combination abolish the
release of free (^{14}C-1)-leucine from labeled protein.
In E. coli B, glucose depletion must be gradual to
stimulate proteolysis; the pool size of several amino
acids then falls significantly. The energy supply is
postulated to regulate intracellular proteolysis indirectly via the RC locus of stringent control.
    Catabolite repression as mediated by cyclic adeno-
sine 3,5-phosphate (cAMP) has no specific influence
on intracellular proteolysis, and proteolysis in a
cAMP-less mutant is normal. A proposed regulation of
intracellular proteolysis by RNA is also discounted.
    On stepwise treatment with toluene, intracellular
proteolysis is first inhibited and then partially re-
appears, producing mostly peptides with molecular
sizes below that of bacitracin. Proteolysis is no
longer affected by energy sources or energy inhibitors.

Other organic solvents also induce incomplete breakdown to peptides. It is proposed that energy is required to render protein substrates accessible for
proteolysis.

Guanosine tetraphosphate, a proposed regulator of
stringent metabolic control does not affect intracellular proteolysis of cells permeabilized by toluenization or cold shock.

Introduction

The metabolic turnover of individual microbial cell
proteins must be determined by a variety of factors.
Only one-fourth of the intracellular protein of E.coli
is subject to breakdown, in distinction to nearly all
the protein of the animal cell (15). The large inac-
cessible remainder, either because of structure or
intracellular localization, cannot be recycled by E.
coli even under prolonged starvation. At the opposite
extreme, a minor population of the cell protein is
rapidly proteolyzed within minutes after synthesis
(14). This may represent either maturation or disposal
of aborted proteins such as has been described here by
Dr. Bukhari, and is fairly constant in rate. The
remaining, slower cell proteolysis is, however, subject to nutritional regulation via the RC gene locus
of stringent control (15,16,17). This general regulatory system stimulates proteolysis and simultaneously
suppresses several biosynthetic pathways in accordance
with the extent of ribosomal idling (3,7). This would
explain the variable proteolytic stimulation by deficiencies of different amino acids (16). Guanosine
tetraphosphate (ppGpp), a factor synthesized by idling
ribosomes, may possibly be the primary mediator of
stringent control (8). One would then expect ppGpp
to stimulate intracellular proteolysis in cells suit-
ably permeabilized to it.

Do other control mechanisms also regulate general
proteolysis? Its rate can be stimulated by energy
deficiency, suggesting the possible role of cyclic
3',5'-adenosine monophosphate (cAMP)-mediated catabolite repression, as has also been suggested here by

Drs. Chang and Goldberg. Energy must in fact have
more than one regulatory role, for its depletion has
been reported to stimulate, inhibit or have no effect
on intracellular proteolysis in different microbial
systems (5,9,10,13,18). In addition, RNA has been
proposed as a proteolytic regulator because its precursors can alter proteolytic rate (18).

These unresolved questions have all been examined
for their bearing on proteolytic regulation. Present
findings suggest that the energy supply controls proteolysis via stringent control rather than catabolite
repression. In addition, there is a second role of
energy as an absolute requirement for intracellular
proteolysis. The effect of RNA precursors is in
reality one of many effects of adenine toxicity. Intracellular proteolysis is not stimulated by ppGpp in
cells permeabilized by cold shock or toluenization.
This at least rules out a role of ppGpp as a direct
feedback effector. When membrane barriers are disrupted by toluenization, an interesting progressive
dissolution of the proteolytic reaction occurs. The
dissociation of proteolysis from its dependence on
energy has been studied further.

Experimental Methods

Intracellular proteolysis was measured as previously
described (15). Cells were labeled with (^{14}C-1)-leu-
cine, filter-washed and resuspended in new medium with
a large excess of leucine-^{12}C. The radioactivity of
free leucine released by proteolysis was recovered by
decarboxylation with ninhydrin. To determine cellular
free amino acid pools with minimal manipulation, 200
ml of culture incubated 30 min in complete or deficient medium was rapidly collected on prewarmed 142
mm diameter cellulose acetate filters, 0.22 μm pore
diameter. Just before the medium had sucked dry, the
membranes were flooded with 10 ml of 10% trichloroacetic acid, and this and two additional washings
were drained and then sucked through the filter. The
combined extracts were deacidified with five ether
extractions, dried and assayed on a Beckman amino acid
analyzer (1).

67

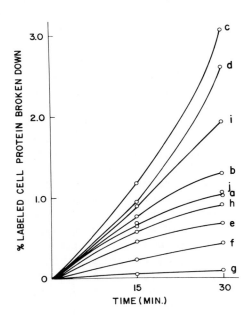

Figure 1: Effect of nutritional deprivation and energy antagonism on intracellular proteolysis in E. coli B in complete and modified medium: (a) complete medium; (b) minus glucose; (c) minus NH₄ and glucose; (e) with 10 mM NaF; (f) 1 mM DNP or (g) DNA and NaF all in complete medium; (h) with NaF; (i) DNP or (j) DNP and NaF all in glucose-free medium.

To permeabilize cells by cold-shock (8), dense suspensions in 0.05M tris (hydroxymethyl)aminomethane HCl, pH 7.9, were sprayed through a fine orifice into 20 volumes of the same buffer plus 1 mM EDTA with rapid stirring, and then supplemented to contain 10 mM $MgCl_2$ 40 mM KCl and 0.1 mM glutathione. Energy was supplied by a mixture of 20 mM ATP, 0.2M phosphoenol pyruvate and 5 μg of pyruvate kinase/ml readjusted to pH 7.9.

In gel filtration experiments, 2 ml of culture was labeled 1 hour with 5-20 μCi of (^{3}H-4,5)-leucine, 30 Ci/mmole, or with 0.5 μCi of (^{14}C-1)-leucine, 50 mCi/mmole. The cells were allowed to proteolyze 1 hour with or without toluenization. The acid-soluble material was deacidified with ether and was applied in 0.05M trimethylamine formate, pH 8.0 to a 61 x 1.5 cm diam. column of Bio-Gel P-2, 200-400 mesh at 0.2 ml/min.

Dr. Michael Cashel, National Institutes of Health, kindly supplied the ppGpp, and Dr. Ira H. Pastan, National Cancer Institute, supplied the cAMP-less mutant and its parent.

Experimental Results

The diverse proteolytic effects of a reduced energy supply can be demonstrated in a single experiment with E. coli B (Fig. 1). When the energy supply is only partly curtailed, proteolysis increases. The increase is slight when glycolysis is inhibited by F or maximal when oxidative phosphorylation is inhibited by 2,4-dinitrophenol (DNP) or when both pathways are inhibited, provided glucose is also present. In the absence of glucose, these inhibitors inhibit proteolysis singly and abolish it in combination. Thus, there is an absolute energy requirement for proteolysis at a low level, but at higher levels the energy supply acts as a negative regulator. In E. coli 9723f (data not shown), proteolysis is also approximately doubled upon inhibition of oxidative phosphorylation with carbonyl cyanide-m-chlorophenylhydrazone (CCCP) at a minimal 2 μM concentration, or upon removal of O_2 by atmospheric evacuation or upon removal of glucose by filter-washing. This last treatment has the same

action in E. coli (Fig. 1). Nath & Koch (10) likewise
found no proteolytic effect of glucose removal in this
strain. There is, however, a proteolytic response to
normal glucose depletion, for upon addition of 2 µg of
glucose/ml, which could last only a few minutes, the
proteolytic rate doubles as in the other strains.
Correspondingly, the cell pool levels of aspartate
plus asparagine, glutamate plus glutamine, glycine,
histidine, valine and threonine all fall. The ratios
of the deficient/normal pool levels (nmol/mg dry cell
weight) are 3.6/8.3; 11/36; 0.85/1.8; 0.16/0.45; 1.1/
4.2; and 0.29/0.59, respectively. These decreases
are significant, for the pool levels of several individual auxotrophic amino acids also fall by half to
three-quarters in cells specifically starved of the
amino acids (unpublished results). Thus, the supply
of several effective amino acid regulators is preferentially exhausted, and stringent control should be
generally expressed. However, without the re-addition
of a trace of glucose, only the comparatively ineffective regulator histidine was found depleted, perhaps
marginally, at 0.27 nmol/mg dry cell weight, while
the pool of a number of other amino acids actually
rose as much as severalfold. Since the ribosomes are
not exhausting amino acid pools, they would appear
limited by the sudden glucose removal at the level of
polypeptide assembly. More specific blockade at this
level, for example by ribosomal poisons, characteris-
tically relaxes the stringent response (4,15,17).
This correlation indicates that the energy supply controls intracellular proteolysis indirectly through
the stringent response via lowering of the pool levels
of a number of amino acids.

No additional regimen, such as the cAMP-mediated
system of catabolite repression (6) appears to be
regulating intracellular proteolysis during energy
restriction. In the Crookes strain of E. coli proteolysis was found unaffected by 3 hours of growth treatment with 1 or 3 mM cAMP, although the growth rate was

TABLE 1

EFFECT OF NUCLEOSIDES ON INTRACELLULAR

PROTEOLYSIS IN E. COLI 9723f phe⁻ thr⁻

Supplements	% Cell protein broken down in 3 h
Complete medium	2.3
-thr	6.5
- " + A	4.4
- " + A, + G, C or U	3.2 - 4.5
- " + A, + G + C, C + U or G + U	4.1 - 4.4
- " + A + G + C + U	4.6
- " + G, C or U	5.7 - 6.1
- " + : G + C, C + U or G + U	5.2 - 5.9
- " + C + G + U	5.5

Thr = threonine, A = adenosine, G = guanosine, C = cytidine, U = uridine all at 100 μg/ml.

approximately halved at either concentration. Also, the proteolytic rate in the cAMP-less mutant 5336 of E. coli K12 (12) was found to closely resemble that of the parent 1100 strain during both growth and starvation of glucose. Again, addition of 3 mM cAMP under either condition had no effect.

Willetts' observed inhibition of proteolysis by RNA precursors (18) could be repeated in E. coli 9723 f, but the effect in essence amounts to an antagonism of stringent control. Thus, in threonine-starved cells, inhibition of proteolysis by any combination of the four precursor nucleosides (Table I) or their free bases (data not shown) could be duplicated by adenosine, which is a growth inhibitor of E. coli and produces a stringent response in RNA synthesis (11). Under these conditions, adenosine regulates ineffectively, and like ineffective amino acid regulators (16) it antagonizes the effective amino acids. Thus, in one experiment adenosine reduced intracellular proteolysis of threonine-starved cells by 33% and simultaneously increased (^{3}H-6)-uracil incorporation 3.5 fold. Adenosine antagonism is limited. It suppressed proteolysis during other amino acid deficiencies or growth on succinate, but not significantly during growth on glucose or starvation of glucose or NH_4^+. Adenine has been reported to inhibit the synthesis of Krebs cycle intermediates and thiamine (11), but additions of succinate or thiamine did not alter proteolytic inhibition by adenosine in threonine-starved cells. In distinction to other studies on adenine toxicity (11) the proteolysis inhibition is demonstrable when growth is already fully inhibited. There appears to be no further basis for considering RNA metabolism to be directly involved in the control of intracellular proteolysis.

Proteolysis in permeabilized cells. Each of the permeabilization treatments examined produces distinctive effects on intracellular proteolysis. Proteolysis in cold-shocked cells is nearly trebled upon the addition of the ATP-generating system but the stimulation occurs after a lag of about 20 min. This may additionally demonstrate a direct energy requirement for proteolysis, but the existence of a lag period makes this interpretation somewhat uncertain. Cold-shocked cells do not synthesize ppGpp endogenously (R. A. Lazzarini, personal communication). The addition of 1 mM ppGpp did not alter either initial or final proteolytic rate.

Emulsification with organic solvents such as ether, chloroform or toluene allows proteolysis at more or less normal initial rates, but the product is mostly acid-soluble material that is not decarboxylated with ninhydrin (Fig. 2; c,d and h). Although the normal product can be judged to be free amino acid on the basis of its susceptibility to decarboxylation (Fig. 2a) and its elution on Bio-Gel P-2 (Fig. 3), in toluenized cells fragments are produced with molecular weights principally below that of bacitracin (1400 daltons). They are peptide in nature for after overnight hydrolysis in 6N HCl the product is virtually completely susceptible to ninhydrin decarboxylation. Intact and toluenized cultures show identical high molecular weight profiles on Sephadex G-100 after they are sonicated and the particulate matter centrifuged out (unpublished experiments). Therefore, the proteolytic attack appears all-or-none with little random breakdown to large fragments. The production of peptides cannot be attributed to loss of energy sources, for intact cells poisoned with DNP and F⁻ still produce free amino acid (Fig. 3). It is therefore likely that disruption of membrane integrity (19) allows low molecular weight peptides to escape from the cell before they can be thoroughly cleaved by final peptidase action. Limited toluenization (Fig. 2; f and g) produces partial effects, including a net inhibition of initial proteolytic cleavage (Fig. 2g). This might be due to early disruption of the energy supply. However, with sufficient toluenization proteolysis must eventually be dissociated from its energy requirement, for the peptonization rate cannot be further altered with either the inhibitors DNP and F⁻ or with glucose or ATP. Again, 1 mM ppGpp is without effect (curves not shown). This would indicate that

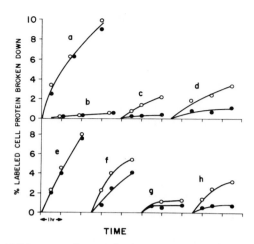

Figure 2: Effect of various treatments on the production of trichloroacetic acid-soluble (0—0) and
ninhydrin-decarboxylated (●—●) radioactivity from
(^{14}C-1)-leucine labelled cell proteins of E. coli
9723f. Expt. a-d, minus glucose and NH_4^+: (a) no
addition, (b) with 1 mM DNP and 10 mM NaF, (c)
emulsified with ether, and (d) emulsified with
chloroform. Expt. e-h, the medium is free of NH_4^+:
(d) no addition, (f) 0.1% toluene, (g) 0.23%
toluene, (h) emulsified with excess toluene.

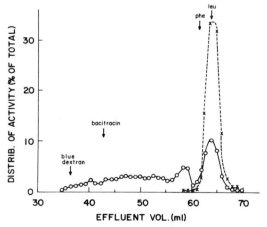

Figure 3: Bio-Gel P-2 gel chromatography of leucine-
labeled trichloroacetic acid-soluble components of
intact (^{14}C)-leucine-labeled (X---X) and toluenized
(^{3}H-4,5)-leucine-labeled (0—0) cells of E. coli
9723f starved of NH_4^+ and glucose. Without trichloroacetic acid, the elution profiles were the same
except for a large protein peak at the exclusion
volume.

when membranes are intact, energy is required to render the protein substrate accessible to the proteolytic apparatus. Similar conclusions have been reached in studies on mammalian cells (2). When cells were protoplasted by 2-1/2 hour exposure to 400 μg penicillin/ml in 18% sucrose, proteolysis dropped to a low rate of 0.2%/hour and was stimulated severalfold when the cells were lysed by resuspension in sucrose-free medium. This may point to an involvement of the periplasmic space in intracellular proteolysis. Although ppGpp could not directly stimulate the proteases of permeabilized cells it is still possible that it controls intracellular proteolysis by more indirect means. Lazzarini & Johnson (8) were likewise unable to show a direct and specific regulation by ppGpp of RNA biosynthesis in cold-shocked E. coli.

References

1. Benson, J. V., Gordon, M. J. & Patterson, J. A. Anal. Biochem. 18, 228 (1967).
2. Brostrom, C. O. & Jeffay, H. J. Biol. Chem. 245, 4001 (1970).
3. Edlin, G. & Broda, P. Bacteriol. Rev. 32, 206 (1969).
4. Goldberg, A. L. Proc. Natl. Acad. Sci. USA 68, 362 (1971).
5. Halvorson, H. O. in Amino Acid Pools (J. T. Holden, ed.) pp. 646-654. Elsevier Publishing Co., Amsterdam (1962).
6. Hardman, J. G. in Cyclic AMP (R. W. Butcher & E. W. Sutherland, ed.) Chapter 12. Academic Press, New York (1971).
7. Haseltine, W. A., Block, R., Gilbert, W. & Weber, K. Nature New Biol. 238, 381 (1972).
8. Lazzarini, R. A. & Johnson, L. D. Nature New Biol. 243, 17 (1973).
9. Mandelstam, J. Biochem. J. 69, 110 (1958).
10. Nath, K. & Koch, A. L. J. Biol. Chem. 246, 6956 (1971).
11. Neidhardt, F. C. Biochim. Biophys. Acta 68, 365 (1963).

12. Perlman, R. L. & Pastan, I. C. Biochem. Biophys. Res. Commun. 37, 151 (1969).
13. Pine, M. J. Biochim. Biophys. Acta 104, 439 (1965).
14. Pine, M. J. J. Bacteriol. 103, 207 (1970).
15. Pine, M. J. J. Bacteriol. 115, 107 (1973).
16. Pine, M. J. J. Bacteriol. 116, 1253 (1973).
17. Sussman, A. J. & Gilvarg, C. J. Biol. Chem. 244, 6304 (1969).
18. Willetts, N. S. Biochem. J. 103, 453 (1967).
19. Woldringh, C. L. J. Bacteriol. 114, 1359 (1973).

ROLE OF ENZYME STABILITY AND TURNOVER IN THE REGULATION OF BIOSYNTHETIC ENZYME LEVELS DURING THE CELL CYCLE OF EUCARYOTIC MICROORGANISMS

Robert R. Schmidt

Department of Biochemistry and Nutrition
Virginia Polytechnic Institute and State University
Blacksburg, Virginia 24061

Introduction

Eucaryotic microorganisms with long cell cycles are confronted with similar problems as the eucaryotic cell in tissues of higher organisms in which cell division occurs infrequently. Both cell types must be able to reduce the levels of certain enzymes in response to environmental change in the absence of frequent cell division. Therefore, it is likely that long-cycled eucaryotic microorganisms, such as Chlorella, have evolved mechanisms for turnover of many enzymes while short-cycled eucaryotic microorganisms, such as the budding and fission yeasts, have not been under selective pressures to evolve mechanisms other than cell division to reduce the levels of unwanted enzymes. However, although many proteins and enzymes in yeasts have been shown (1,2,3) to be stable in exponentially growing cells, there are probably mechanisms for controlling the turnover of key regulatory enzymes during the normal cell cycle and also mechanisms for degrading many proteins for cell maintenance during the stationary phase of non-growing cells.

One of the research objectives in this laboratory has been to use synchronous cultures of the highly compartmentalized eucaryotic microorganism, Chlorella,

as a model system to study regulation of enzyme levels
during the cell cycle of eucaryotic cells. From certain types of enzyme patterns obtained in cell cycle
studies, it is possible to make predictions regarding
the role of enzyme-stability, turnover, and gene dosage effects on regulation of enzyme levels during the
cell cycle. The present chapter will concern the
regulation of a number of biosynthetic enzymes, whereas
a recent review (4) discusses studies from this laboratory on regulation of inducible enzymes during the cell
cycle of this eucaryote.

Models for Regulation of Enzyme Accumulation During Eucaryotic Cell Cycles

Although considerable experimental evidence supports
the model that synthesis of biosynthetic enzymes is
regulated by oscillatory repression (5,6) during the
cell cycle of procaryotes, there is a scarcity of evidence to support the oscillatory repression model or
any other model for cell cycle regulation of levels
of biosynthetic enzymes in eucaryotic cells. This
lack of understanding of cell cycle controls in eucaryotes stems from the greater number of possible
options that must be considered in interpreting enzyme
patterns and other cell cycle data from eucaryotes.
Higher eucaryotic plant (7) and animal (8-11) cells
differ from the procaryotes in that a number of post-
transcriptional events (e.g., processing of precursor
mRNA, transport of mRNA from nucleus to cytoplasm,
stability of mRNA, enzyme turnover, etc.) are more
likely to obscure the timing between gene transcription and enzyme synthesis or accumulation during the
cell cycle. Schmidt (4) has recently discussed in
more detail these and other post-transcriptional factors which complicate interpretation of studies on
regulation of enzyme levels in eucaryotes.

A restricted gene-transcription model has been
proposed (12,13) which predicts that differences in
the timing of accumulation of different biosynthetic
enzymes results from a sequential transcription of the
genome during the cell cycle. In this model, specific

78

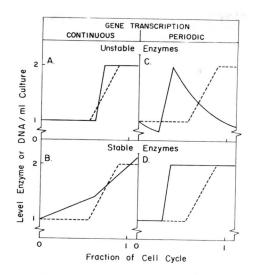

Figure 1: Predicted patterns for biosynthetic enzymes, stable or unstable _in vivo_ with their genes transcribed continuously or periodically, during the cell cycle of synchronous eucaryotic cells. ——— and -----, enzyme and DNA levels, respectively. mRNA assumed to be labile and post-transcriptional factors non-limiting throughout the cell cycle. Patterns from Schmidt (4).

genes are visualized as being transcribed only at given times in the eucaryotic cell cycle. In view of recent findings of post-transcriptional mechanisms in eucaryotes, this model could be modified by proposing some periodic post-transcriptional event such as periodic processing of precursor mRNA or periodic transport of mRNA from the nucleus, instead of periodic transcription.

The oscillatory repression model (5,6) predicts that genes are continuously available for transcription throughout the cell cycle. Periodic enzyme accumulation is visualized as resulting from the operation of feedback repression circuits in which the enzyme and corepressor (e.g., pathway end-product) form part of a closed feedback system in which the concentration of one determines the rate of synthesis of the other. As a result of these interactions, the cellular concentration of both enzyme and corepressor oscillates. Since inducible biosynthetic enzymes must also be considered in eucaryotes, the model might be more appropriately called the oscillatory repression-induction model.

What types of enzyme patterns are predicted for biosynthetic enzymes regulated by either of these proposed mechanisms? The restricted gene-transcription mechanism predicts that only during periods in which a gene is accessible for transcription would the typical Jacob-Monod type of regulation of gene activity be operative. In this situation, step patterns (Fig. 1D) are predicted for stable enzymes, and periodic patterns (Fig. 1C) are predicted for unstable enzymes during the cell cycle. Moreover, linear enzyme patterns would not be observed. Although it can be argued that a mechanism of this type can order the sequence of biochemical events required to program the cell's development through the cell cycle, it can also be argued that a cell's biosynthetic system cannot readily respond to changes in the external environment under such a mechanism of control.

If genes are continuously accessible for transcription, as proposed in the oscillatory repression-induction

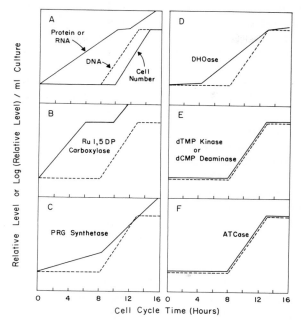

Figure 2: Patterns for total protein, RNA, DNA, cell
number and six different biosynthetic enzymes during the cell cycle of Chlorella pyrenoidosa (strain
7-11-05) under constant environmental conditions.
(A). Log (relative level total protein, RNA, DNA,
and cell number); Relative levels: (B) Ribulose
1,5-diphosphate carboxylase; (C) Phosphoribosyl
glycinamide synthetase; (D) Dihydroorotase; (E)
dTMP kinase or dCMP deaminase; (F) Aspartate
transcarbamylase; ----, DNA level.

model, a number of different patterns of accumulation
of biosynthetic enzymes are possible during the cell
cycle. If the level of repression is constant (i.e.,
corepressor or inducer not oscillating), a stable enzyme should accumulate in a linear manner (Fig. 1B)
with a change in rate of linear accumulation occurring
at the time of gene replication, whereas an unstable
enzyme is predicted to accumulate in a step pattern
(Fig. 1A) with the step-increase also occurring within
the S-phase. When an unstable enzyme is not accumulating under these conditions, a steady state will
exist between synthesis and breakdown of the enzyme.
Mutations which result in constitutive synthesis of
stable and unstable enzymes will generate patterns
identical to those predicted for conditions in which
the level of repression is constant. When the level
of repression (or induction) is oscillating (in the
wild-type), the patterns of both stable and unstable
enzymes will approach step patterns, and these steps
can presumably occur at any time in the cell cycle
(see ref. 4 for additional discussion).

Regulation of Levels of Biosynthetic Enzymes During
the Chlorella Cell Cycle

The cell cycle of strain 7-11-05 of C. pyrenoidosa
is characterized (14) by a long G1-phase, an S-phase
near the end of the cell cycle, and a short G2-phase
(Fig. 2A). Total protein and RNA increase exponentially with the same exponential coefficient during
the cell cycle (Fig. 2A). These macromolecular fractions cease to increase for a short time interval following the onset of DNA replication. This period of
reduced accumulation is usually seen (14) in synchronous cells selected by equilibrium centrifugation (15,
16) from asynchronous cultures growing in continuous
light; it is often not apparent in light-dark syn-
chronized cells. Since many enzymes are synthesized
and accumulate during this period, does this period
reflect a reduced rate of synthesis of ribosomal RNA
and structural proteins?

82

Biosynthetic enzymes are observed to accumulate in step patterns during the cell cycles of most eucaryotic microorganisms (17,18). However, the strain of Chlorella used in this laboratory appears to be an exception in that linear and step patterns are observed for biosynthetic enzymes in this eucaryotic microorganism (Fig. 2B,C,D,E,F). Moreover, these linear and step patterns are exhibited by both stable and unstable enzymes (in vivo) during the cell cycle.

Ribulose-1,5-Diphosphate Carboxylase. The first evidence that a structural gene of a biosynthetic enzyme is continuously available for transcription and that enzyme turnover plays an important role in regulating enzyme levels during the cell cycle of this eucaryote came from studies with ribulose-1,5-diphosphate carboxylase (Fig. 2B). The pattern of this enzyme could be changed from a step to a continuous pattern merely by increasing the growth rate of the organism (19). Moreover, when added at any time during the cell cycle, inhibitors of protein (i.e, cycloheximide) and RNA (i.e., actinomycin D or azaserine) synthesis blocked carboxylase accumulation and the enzyme activity decayed in a first order manner with a half-life of 4.4 hours (20). Under conditions in which enzyme accumulation is periodic, inhibitor studies indicate that a steady state exists between carboxylase synthesis and breakdown during the period of constant activity between the sixth and ninth hours of the cell cycle. Thus, rather than an on-off mechanism of gene transcription resulting in periodic enzyme accumulation, a changing rate of transcription and a constant rate of enzyme turnover appear to regulate the level of the carboxylase during the cell cycle. The initial step-increase in the carboxylase occurs outside of the S-phase. As stated in an earlier section of this chapter, the step-increase in an unstable enzyme can occur outside the S-phase if the level of corepressor is oscillating.

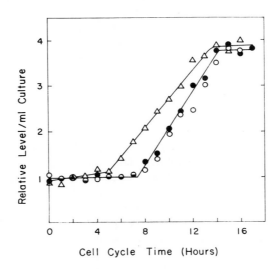

Figure 3: Relative levels of aspartate transcarbamylase (0), dihydroorotase (Δ), and DNA (0) during the
cell cycle of Chlorella pyrenoidosa (strain 7-11-05)
under constant environmental conditions. Dunn &
Schmidt (22).

Phosphoribosylglycinamide Synthetase. Phosphoribosylglycinamide synthetase, the second enzyme on the
purine biosynthetic pathway, was observed (21) to
increase in a linear manner with a change in rate of
linear accumulation occurring at the onset of the
period of DNA replication (Fig. 2C). The level of
the enzyme remained constant for a 6-hour period (in
vivo) in which total protein and RNA synthesis were
inhibited in separate cell cycle experiments. Thus,
the linear pattern of this stable enzyme and its change
in rate of linear accumulation within the period of DNA
replication provides evidence that the structural gene
of this enzyme is transcribed continuously and is either
free from repression or is under essentially a constant
level of repression during the cell cycle.

Dihydroorotase. Although the stable phosphoribosylglycinamide synthetase accumulates in a linear manner
throughout the cell cycle, another stable (in vivo)
enzyme, dihydroorotase, was recently observed by Dunn
& Schmidt (22) to accumulate in essentially a periodic
manner during the Chlorella cell cycle (Fig. 2D,3).
Cycloheximide has been shown to inhibit the step increase indihydroorotase activity and the enzyme activity does not decay in a subsequent 3- to 4-hour period in the presence of the inhibitor. The step-
increase in activity begins outside the period of DNA
replication and the rate of increase in enzyme activity differs from that of the DNA (Fig. 3), indicating
that the increase in enzyme activity is not directly
coupled to gene replication. In the three cell cycle
experiments in which the level of the enzyme has been
measured, there appears to be a slow accumulation of
the enzyme before and after the major step in enzyme
activity. This gradual increase in activity is predicted for a stable enzyme whose synthesis is being
controlled by oscillatory-repression or induction.
In the oscillatory repression-induction model, the
binding of corepressor (or inducer) with the aporepres-
sor (or repressor) is assumed to be reversible as is
the repressor-operator interaction (23). The rate of
transcription and thereby the rate of enzyme synthesis

will approach zero asymptotically, but will never become zero. Thus, when a corepressor (or inducer) is oscillating and the gene dosage remains constant, a stable enzyme will accumulate at a low rate whereas the level of an unstable enzyme will remain constant between the major bursts of enzyme accumulation.

dTMP Kinase and dCMP Deaminase. In earlier publications (24,25) from this laboratory, the patterns of dCMP deaminase and dTMP kinase, two enzymes on the dTTP biosynthetic pathway, were expressed on a specific activity basis (i.e., percentage of total cellular-P or cell volume) and compared to the DNA pattern. The patterns of these enzymes were essentially identical during the last half of the cell cycle. Moreover, although the enzyme patterns were similar to the DNA pattern, the peak in specific activity of DNA was displaced about 1 to 1.5 hours later in the cell cycle from the peak in specific activity of these enzymes. Because of incomplete extraction of DNA from cells early in the cell cycle and certain non-DNA substances which increased near the end of the cell cycle which contributed chromophores in the procedure used to analyze for DNA, the DNA pattern reported in these early studies (26) recently was shown (14) to be incorrect. When the patterns of these two enzymes are expressed on a per ml of culture basis and compared to a corrected DNA pattern expressed on the same basis, the enzyme and DNA patterns are essentially coincident during the S-phase (Fig. 2E). Wanka & Poels (27) observed the levels (per ml of culture) of dTMP kinase and uridine kinase to remain constant and then to increase in coincident fashion with the step-increase in DNA in another strain (211-8b) of C. pyrenoidosa.

The essentially identical timing of the step-increases in these nucleotide biosynthetic enzymes and the step-increase in DNA is consistent with the model of regulation predicted for unstable enzymes whose structural genes are expressed continuously and are either free from repression or under a constant level of repression during the cell cycle (Fig. 1A). When the rate of protein synthesis in strain 7-11-05 is slowed either by placing the cells under a reduced light intensity or in the dark, the levels of these enzymes decrease. Wanka & Poels (27) have also observed the level of dTMP kinase to decay in cells of strain 211-8b placed in the dark. Before it can be ascertained whether or not the patterns of these enzymes reflect the continuous synthesis of enzymes which turn over continuously throughout the cell cycle, detailed turnover studies will be required at different times in the cell cycle. The possibility exists that the enzyme and DNA patterns are identical because the structural genes of these enzymes only become available for transcription immediately prior to or after replication in the S-phase.

Aspartate Transcarbamylase. The pattern of accumulation of aspartate transcarbamylase, the first enzyme on the pyrimidine biosynthetic pathway, was reported by Vassef et al. (28) to be very similar to the pattern for DNA except for a period of gradual enzyme accumulation immediately prior to the step-increase in DNA. However, very recent experiments in this laboratory (Dunn & Schmidt [22]) have shown the patterns of the enzyme and DNA to be coincident (Fig. 2F,3).

Because the relative increase in the enzyme level always exceeded that of the DNA or cell number during each cell cycle, the enzyme patterns reported earlier (28) should have been recognized sooner as being incorrect. All parameters must increase in direct relation to the cell number or DNA during a cell cycle of balanced synchronous growth. Other parameters and experiments indicated that these synchronous cells exhibited balanced synchronous growth. Thus, the greater fold-increase in enzyme was proposed to be due to either a low recovery of enzyme at the beginning of the cell cycle or an excess recovery (or synthesis) of the enzyme near the end of the cell cycle. The former appears to be true. Although samples harvested at different times in the cell cycle were thawed for a constant period of time prior to assay, more of the enzyme decayed during the thawing process in samples harvested from the first 5 hours of the cell cycle than in samples from 5 to 10 hours in the cell cycle. An endogenous stabilizer (28) of the enzyme appears to increase during the 4- to 5-hour period immediately preceding and for a time during the S-phase and to protect the enzyme from decay in vitro prior to assay. By freezing and thawing all harvest samples in the presence of 2 mM uridine, it has been possible to stabilize the enzyme and to prevent its decay in all harvest samples. (Freezing and thawing Chlorella cells once at -20° breaks permeability barriers to small molecules and permits assay of enzymes within the thawed cells.) When the enzyme is stabilized in vitro prior to assay, its pattern is essentially coincident with that of DNA during the cell cycle (Fig. 3).

The pattern of accumulation of the enzyme is consistent with that of an unstable enzyme which is synthesized continuously and whose structural gene is either free from repression or under a constant level of repression during the cell cycle. If the enzyme is unstable in vivo and its structural gene regulated as stated, the following relationships should exist: (a) a modified DNA pattern should give rise to a similarly modified enzyme pattern, (b) a steady state between enzyme synthesis and degradation should exist during periods of constant enzyme activity, and (c) the enzyme should be unstable at all times during the cell cycle.

The step DNA pattern can be modified to a semi-continuous pattern by increasing the light intensity continuously during the cell cycle. When DNA accumulated in this semi-continuous pattern, the enzyme pattern paralleled that of the DNA, suggesting that a direct relationship might exist between gene replication and accumulation of the enzyme (28).

When either cycloheximide or actinomycin D was added to synchronously growing cells during the first 4 hours of the cell cycle, a rapid decay in aspartate transcarbamylase activity was observed (28). This observation is consistent with the interpretation that

a steady state between synthesis and breakdown exists
during periods of constant activity. Since the enzyme
and DNA patterns are coincident and the enzyme appears
to turn over during periods of constant activity, one
would predict that the enzyme would also turn over
during the period of the step-increase in enzyme activity. However, when cycloheximide was added to synchronously growing cells at 9.5 hours of the cell cycle,
the increase in enzyme activity was blocked, but the
enzyme activity did not decay as seen early in the cell
cycle. At present, there is no explanation for this
apparent paradox. Perhaps the cells are less permeable
to cycloheximide later in the cell cycle and a higher
concentration of the inhibitor is needed to totally
block enzyme synthesis. Thus, final conclusions
regarding the in vivo turnover of the enzyme must
await additional turnover studies with cycloheximide
and other inhibitors and the use of a more direct procedure, such as a radioimmunoprecipitin procedure, to
evaluate the problem of aspartate transcarbamylase
turnover at different times in the cell cycle.

The enzyme is stable in concentrated cell homogenates prepared from cells at the tenth hour of the
cell cycle. Removal of an endogenous stabilizer from
these homogenates by either ultrafiltration, gel filtration, ammonium sulfate precipitation, or sucrose
density-gradient centrifugation results in the rapid
first-order decay of the enzyme at 0-3° (28). Properties of the endogenous stabilizer are: (a) complete stability at 100° at pH 9.2 for at least 15 min;
(b) molecular weight less than 1000; (c) adsorbable
to Norit-A; (d) no retention to a cation-exchange
resin at pH 3.0; and (e) destroyed by ashing. Since
ashing destroys the stabilizer, it is not likely a
metal ion. Since the endogenous stabilizer is heat
stable and is not retained by a cation exchange at
low pH, it cannot be one of the substrates of the
enzyme, carbamyl phosphate, or aspartate (or most
other amino acids or peptides), respectively.

After passage of an acidified extract through a
cation-exchange column (Dowex-50, x-4, H^+ form, 200-

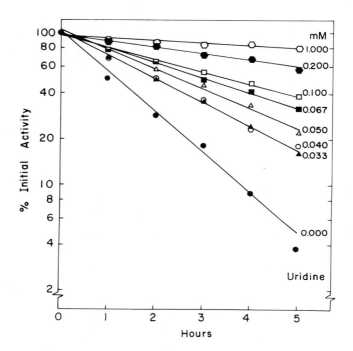

Figure 4: In vitro decay of Chlorella aspartate
transcarbamylase activity at 0-3° in the presence
of different concentrations of uridine. For decay
studies, the enzyme was dissolved in 0.2M Tris-HCl
buffer (pH 8.5, containing 1 mM EDTA) after precipitation with 50 to 70% ammonium sulfate from
100,000 x g supernatant of a cell homogenate.
Wilkins & Schmidt (30).

300 mesh), the eluate contained only two UV-absorbing (254 nm) peaks as determined by high pressure liquid chromatography (29). The position of these peaks corresponded to uridine and UMP. We have tested (28) most of the commonly occurring bases, nucleosides, and nucleotides (mono-, di-, and triphosphates) for their ability to stabilize aspartate transcarbamylase. Only uridine and UMP, which are potent inhibitors of the enzyme, are effective stabilizers (28).

Although uridine and UMP are in high enough concentration (approx. 0.2 to 0.2 mM) to stabilize the enzyme in these homogenates, there may be other endogenous stabilizer(s) which are not UV-absorbing and have gone undetected so far. The identification of all possible endogenous stabilizers requires the development of a quantitative procedure for determining the stabilizer concentration in cell homogenates, fractions from columns, etc. Furthermore, a reproducible procedure for measuring the rate of enzyme decay is also essential for evaluating other factors affecting the rate of decay of aspartate transcarbamylase activity.

Wilkins and Schmidt (30) have recently developed a procedure for quantifying the effects of stabilizers on the rate of decay of the enzyme. The enzyme is recovered from 100,000 x g supernatants of Chlorella homogenates in a 50 to 70% ammonium sulfate cut. The enzyme is reconstituted in 0.2M Tris-HCl buffer, pH 8.5, containing 2 mM uridine, and the enzyme is stored as a stable preparation. Prior to use in a decay study the enzyme is precipitated from the uridine buffer with 70% ammonium sulfate and then reconstituted in buffer in the absence of uridine. To this enzyme preparation different concentrations of stabilizer are added. Figure 4 shows the different rates of decay of the ammonium sulfate fractionated enzyme at different concentrations of added uridine. The rate constants for decay, k_d, at each uridine concentration are determined from the slopes in these log plots. If the rate constant for decay in the absence of uridine is defined as k_{d_0} and the rate of decay at any given concentration of uridine is defined as k_{d_x}, then a plot of $k_{d_0} - k_{d_x}$

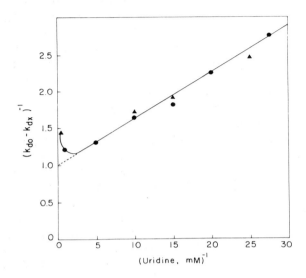

Figure 5: In vitro stability of Chlorella aspartate transcarbamylase activity at 0-3° in the presence of different concentrations of uridine. k_{d_0} and k_{d_x}, rate constants for decay in the absence of uridine and at any given concentration of uridine, respectively. ●, Data from Fig. 4; ▲, data from a replicate experiment. Wilkins & Schmidt (30).

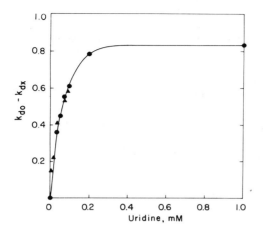

Figure 6: Double reciprocal plot relating the _in vitro_ stability of <u>Chlorella</u> aspartate transcarbamylase activity at 0-3° to uridine concentration. Data from Fig. 5. Wilkins & Schmidt (30).

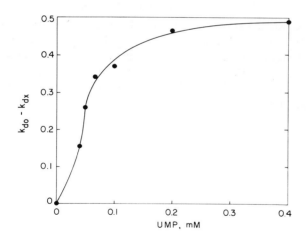

Figure 7: _In vitro_ stability of <u>Chlorella</u> aspartate transcarbamylase activity at 0-3° in the presence of different concentrations of UMP. Conditions and definitions described in Fig. 4 and 5, respectively. Wilkins & Schmidt (30).

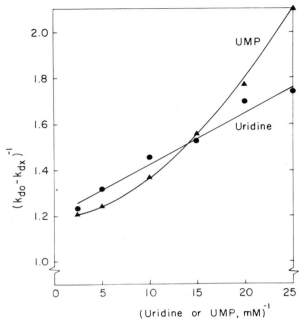

Figure 8: Comparison of the double reciprocal plots for the in vitro stability of Chlorella aspartate transcarbamylase activity at 0–3° in the presence of uridine and UMP. Conditions and definitions described in Figs. 4 and 5, respectively. Wilkins & Schmidt (30).

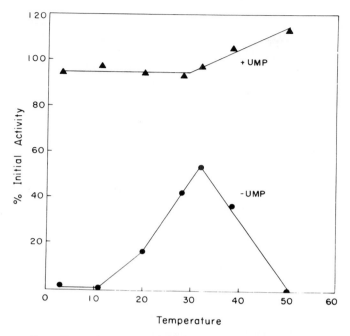

Figure 9: <u>In vitro</u> stability of <u>Chlorella</u> aspartate
transcarbamylase activity at different temperatures
in the presence of 0.4 mM UMP. The stability studies
were performed with whole cells frozen (-20°) and
thawed once to break permeability barriers to small
molecules. The buffer was described in Fig. 4.
The enzyme was maintained at each temperature for
90 min prior to assay. Wilkins & Schmidt (30).

vs. concentration of uridine gives a hyperbolic plot (Fig. 5). A double reciprocal plot indicated that the uridine data could be linearized for use as a standard curve for quantifying the amount of stabilizer in a given preparation (Fig. 6). However, UMP showed cooperative effects on a stabilization of the enzyme (Fig. 7), yielding a nonlinear double reciprocal plot (Fig. 8). Similar cooperative effects were observed in enzyme activity inhibition studies with UMP (28). Maximum stability of the enzyme is reached at approximately 0.4 mM UMP or uridine; however, significant inhibition of enzyme activity is not reached until 0.5 mM uridine and 1 mM UMP (28). The enzyme is stabilized by 0.4 mM UMP over a wide temperature range (Fig. 9). Although the enzyme is unstable in the absence of UMP at all the temperatures tested, it is more stable at 32° than at other temperatures in the absence of UMP.

If the enzyme is in the same cellular compartment with UMP (or uridine), these data provide evidence that a feedback inhibitor might plan an important role in regulating both the level and activity of the first enzyme on a biosynthetic pathway in a eucaryotic cell. In other words, since the enzyme can be stabilized by low concentrations of UMP which are not inhibitory, this nucleotide could act potentially as both a positive and negative regulatory of pyrimidine nucleotide biosynthesis during the cell cycle. Low concentrations of UMP could lead to stabilization of the unstable enzyme and accelerated UMP synthesis, whereas high concentrations of UMP could lead to feedback inhibition of enzyme activity and reduced UMP synthesis.

Recent studies have been aimed at determining the state of repression of the aspartate transcarbamylase gene and also the effects of exogenous uracil and uridine on the pattern of accumulation of the enzyme during the cell cycle of Chlorella. In other eucaryotic microorganisms, such as Saccharomyces cerevisiae and Neurospora crassa, this enzyme is reported to be regulated by repression with pyrimidine nucleotide

endproduct(s). Moreover, a concentration of 0.20 mM
uracil in the culture medium completely inhibited the
accumulation of this enzyme within a single cell cycle
of Bacillus subtilis W3 (31,32).

Chlorella cells cultured for as long as four con-
secutive generations in the presence of 0.267 mM uracil
contained essentially the same level of the enzyme per
cell as control cultures. The uracil was absorbed and
metabolized at this concentration because it had the
ability to restore RNA synthesis to the control value
after RNA synthesis was completely inhibited by addition of 6-azauracil to the culture medium (33). Dunn
& Schmidt (22) have recently shown that a concentration of 40 mM uridine in the culture medium was required
before uridine incorporation into total RNA was constant
in a 1-hour incorporation period in the absence of 6-
azauracil in the culture medium. In these studies,
radioactive uridine was employed. After a 1-hour
incorporation period, 15% of the radioactivity was
associated with the nucleic acid fraction and 85% was
associated with the acid soluble fraction of the cells.
If all of the acid-soluble radioactivity was associated
with uridine, its intracellular concen-ration would be
1.98 mM. Similar incorporation patterns were obtained
with uracil except that a plateau in rate of incorporation into nucleic acid was never reached because of
solubility problems over 29 mM. When synchronous
Chlorella cells were cultured in the presence of 40 mM
uridine for one cell cycle, the patterns of accumulation of aspartate transcarbamylase, dihydroorotase,
total protein, and DNA were identical to those in the
control culture. Is the structural gene of the enzyme
expressed constitutively or is it already expressed at
its basal level because of repressive endogenous levels
of pyrimidine endproducts throughout the cell cycle?
Is the absorbed uridine converted to the true corepressor at a sufficient rate to lead to repressive levels
of the corepressor? Because of cellular compartmen-
talization, is the absorbed uridine and its metabolic
products in equilibrium with the endogenous pyrimidine
nucleotide pool? These are but a few of the pertinent

97

questions that must be answered before it will be possible to determine how the levels of aspartate transcarbamylase are regulated during the cell cycle of
this eucaryote.

Summary

The genes for both stable and unstable biosynthetic
enzymes appear to be continuously available for transcription during the cell cycle of the highly compartmentalized eucaryotic microorganism, Chlorella. There
is no evidence so far to indicate that transcription
of genes of biosynthetic enzymes is restricted to
specific periods of the cell cycle. By changing the
culture conditions during synchronous growth, it has
been possible to change step patterns to continuous
patterns and vice versa. These results coupled with
studies with inhibitors of protein and RNA synthesis
indicate that gene transcription is responsive to the
cell's environment. The genes of a number of biosynthetic enzymes appear to be either free from repression (e.g., expressed constitutively) or under a constant level of repression so that the in vivo stability
of these enzymes and the gene dosage regulates the
pattern of accumulation of these enzymes.

Acknowledgement

The research discussed in this chapter has been
supported by grants from the National Science Foundation (GB17305) and the National Institutes of Health
(GM19871).

References

1. Halvorson, H. O. Biochim. Biophys. Acta 27,
    267 (1958).
2. Mitchison, J. M. & Creanor, J. J. Cell Sci. 5,
    373 (1969).
3. Sebastian, J., Carter, B. L. A., and Halvorson,
    H. O. Eur. J. Biochem. 37, 516 (1973).
4. Schmidt, R. R., in Cell Cycle Controls (G. M.
    Padilla, I. L. Cameron, and A. M. Zimmerman,
    eds.) Academic Press, New York (1974).

5. Donachi, W. D. & Masters, M., in The Cell Cycle: Gene-Enzyme Interactions (G. M. Padilla, G. L. Whitson and I. L. Cameron, eds.), Academic Press, New York (1969) p. 37.
6. Goodwin, B. C. Nature 209, 479 (1966).
7. Zielke, H. R. & Filner, P. J. Biol. Chem. 246, 1772 (1971).
8. Schimke, R. T., in Current Topics in Cell Regulation (B. C. Horecker and B. R. Stadtman, eds.), Vol. I, Academic Press, New York (1969) p. 77.
9. Schimke, R. T. & Doyle, D. Ann. Rev. Biochem. 39, 939 (1970).
10. Darnell, J. E., Jelinek, W. R. & Molloy, G. R. Science 181, 1215 (1973).
11. Kwan, S-W. & Brawerman, G. Proc. Nat. Acad. Sci. U.S.A. 69, 3247 (1972).
12. Halvorson, H. O., Bock, R. M., Tauro, P., Epstein, R. & LaBerge, M. in Cell Synchrony--Studies in Biosynthetic Regulation (I. L. Cameron & G. M. Padilla, eds.), Academic Press, New York (1966), p. 102.
13. Tauro, P. & Halvorson, H. O. J. Bacteriol. 92, 652 (1966).
14. Hopkins, H. A., Flora, J. B. & Schmidt, R. R. Arch. Biochem. Biophys. 153, 845 (1972).
15. Sitz, T. O., Kent, A. B., Hopkins, H. A. & Schmidt, R. R. Science 168, 1231 (1970).
16. Hopkins, H. A., Sitz, T. O. & Schmidt, R. R. J. Cell Physiol. 76, 231 (1970).
17. Mitchison, J. M. Science 165, 657 (1969).
18. Halvorson, H. O., Carter, B. L. A. & Tauro, P. Adv. Microb. Physiol. 6, 47 (1970).
19. Molloy, G. R. & Schmidt, R. R. Biochem. Biophys. Res. Commun. 40, 1125 (1970).
20. Sitz, T. O., Molloy, G. R. & Schmidt, R. R. Biochim. Biophys. Acta 319, 103 (1973).
21. Molloy, G. R., Sitz, T. O. & Schmidt, R. R. J. Biol. Chem. 248, 1970 (1973).
22. Dunn, J. H. & Schmidt, R. R. J. Biol. Chem., in preparation.

23. Bourgeois, S., in Current Topics in Cellular Regulation (B. L. Horecker and E. R. Stadtman, eds.), Vol. 4, Academic Press, New York (1971) p. 39.

24. Shen, S. R–C. & Schmidt, R. R.   Arch. Biochem. Biophys. 115, 13 (1966).

25. Johnson, R. & Schmidt, R. R.   Biochim. Biophys. Acta 129, 140 (1966).

26. Herrmann, E. C. & Schmidt, R. R.   Biochim. Biophys. Acta 95, 63 (1965).

27. Wanka, F. & Poels, C. L. M.   Eur. J. Biochem. 9, 478 (1969).

28. Vassef, A. A., Flora, J. B., Weeks, J. G., Bibbs, B. S. & Schmidt, R. R.   J. Biol. Chem. 248, 1976 (1973).

29. Henry, R. A., Schmit, J. A. & Williams, R. C. J. Chrom. Sci. 11, 358 (1973).

30. Wilkins, J. & Schmidt, R. R.   J. Biol. Chem. in preparation.

31. Donachi, W. D. Nature 205, 1084 (1965).

32. Masters, M. & Donachie, W. E. Nature 209, 476 (1966).

33. Flora, J. B., Ph.D. Dissertation, Virginia Polytechnic Institute, Blacksburg, Virginia (1969).

Regulation of Enzyme Levels
in Animal Tissues

INDUCTION, INTRACELLULAR TRANSFER, AND TURNOVER OF δ-AMINOLEVULINATE SYNTHETASE IN LIVER

Goro Kikuchi, Norio Hayashi, Akira Ohashi,
Haeng Ja Kim and Keiko Watarai

Department of Biochemistry
Tohoku University School of Medicine
Sendai 980, Japan

δ-Aminolevulinate (ALA) synthetase is a key enzyme in the regulation of porphyrin synthesis and this enzyme is usually confined to the mitochondria. The activity of ALA synthetase in liver can be increased greatly by the administration of various drugs such as allylisopropylacetamide (AIA) and 3,5-dicarbethoxy-1,4-dihydrocollidine (1). Previously we demonstrated that in animals treated with AIA a considerable amount of ALA synthetase appeared in not only the mitochondria but also the cytosol fraction (2,3). Studies with cycloheximide and chloramphenicol indicated that both enzymes in the cytosol and the mitochondria are synthesized originally on cytoribosomes (3). Kinetic study of the increase and decrease of ALA synthetase in the different subcellular fractions, as well as the properties of the two ALA synthetases, suggested that the ALA synthetase in the cytosol fraction could be a precursor of mitochondrial ALA synthetase. In the present paper we wish to discuss the induction, intracellular transfer and turnover of ALA synthetase mainly in rat liver.

Methods

Wistar strain male albino rats were fasted for 24-40 hours, after which AIA was administered by subcutaneous injection usually at a dose of 25 mg per 100 g body weight of rats. Subcellular fractions of the

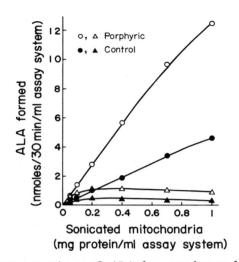

Figure 1: Formation of ALA by sonicated liver mitochondria from control (closed figures) and porphyric
rats (open figures). Reaction mixtures contained
in a final volume of 1 ml: 100 μmoles of Tris–HCl
buffer (pH 7.4), 100 μmoles of glycine, 5 or 0.05
μmoles of ^{14}C-labeled succinate (1 or 10 mCi/mmole,
respectively), 20 μmole of ATP, 10 μmoles of $MgCl_2$,
5 μmoles of EDTA, 0.2 μmoles of pyridoxal phosphate,
0.1 μmole of CoA, 2.5 μg of antimycin A, 5 μmoles
of malonate, 5 units of succinyl–CoA synthetase,
and indicated amounts of sonicated liver mitochondria. Incubation: 30 min at 37°. Radioactive ALA
was isolated as ALA–pyrrole and assayed as described
in Ref. (6). 0, ●: with 5 mM succinate; Δ, ▲: with
0.05 mM succinate.

liver were prepared as described previously (4). The homogenate was centrifuged for 10 min at 600 g and only the supernatant fraction was used in the present study, although a considerable amount of mitochondria precipitated on centrifugation at 600 g. The mitochondria were precipitated by centrifuging the 600 g supernatant for 10 min at 8000 g, and the resulting supernatant was used as the cytosol fraction.

The activity of ALA synthetase was assayed colorimetrically or radiochemically. Assay conditions are given in respective figures. The mitochondrial fraction or liver homogenate were frozen once and thawed or sonicated to ensure the full activity of ALA synthetase (cf. 4,5). Also the assay systems contained a sufficient amount of succinyl-CoA synthetase preparation prepared from Escherichia coli (5) to regenerate and maintain a high level of succinyl-CoA during the reaction. Enzyme activities estimated by the colorimetric and radiochemical assay methods were in good agreement regardless of the amount of mitochondria used. However, to obtain reliable data with either the colorimetric or radiochemical assay, it was important to use large amounts of both succinate and ATP. For instance, when 0.05 mM succinate or 1 mM ATP was employed for the reaction, the activities obtained were far lower than the values obtained by employing 5-10 mM succinate and 10-20 mM ATP, respectively, and as shown in Fig. 1, when 0.05 mM succinate was used as the ^{14}C-labeled substrate, the activity of ALA synthetase in the sonicated liver mitochondria was not proportional to added protein, even in the presence of 20 mM ATP, although the activity in the porphyric rat was definitely higher than that in the control rat. This is probably because the level of succinyl-CoA becomes rate-limiting in the overall reaction of ALA synthesis. When 5 mM succinate was employed, however, a quite reasonable relationship was obtained between the enzyme activity and the amount of protein, and the activity of ALA synthetase in porphyric animals was much higher than the activity in the control animals.

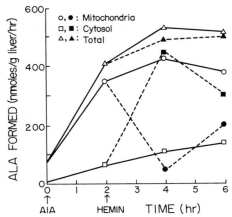

Figure 2: Rats were given hemin (0.5 mg/100 g body weight) i.v., 2 hr after the administration of AIA and killed 0, 2 and 4 hr later. The activity of ALA synthetase was assayed colorimetrically under the conditions described in (4). Open symbols, AIA alone; solid symbols, AIA and hemin.

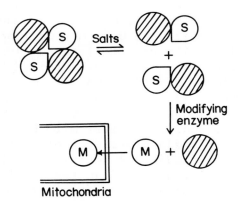

Figure 3: A hypothetical model of the conversion of the cytosol ALA synthetase to the mitochondrial ALA synthetase.

Results and Discussion

Previously we showed that the molecular size of ALA synthetase in the cytosol fraction of rat liver was much larger than that of the mitochondrial ALA synthetase (2). When estimated by gel filtration, the apparent molecular weight of the cytosol ALA synthetase was 600,000, while that of the mitochondrial enzyme was about 115,000. When examined by sucrose density gradient centrifugation, however, the molecular weight of the cytosol ALA synthetase appeared to be about 178,000 while the mitochondrial ALA synthetase again gave 115,000 (2). It seems likely that the cytosol enzyme is bound to a lipoprotein. Also, there was a big difference between their half lives; the apparent half life of the cytosol enzyme was as short as 20 min, while that of the mitochondrial enzyme was about 60 min (3).

It is well known that the induction of ALA synthetase is strongly suppressed by the administration of hemin. However, we found that when hemin was injected to the rats pre-treated with AIA, a large amount of ALA synthetase accumulated in the cytosol fraction, whereas the enzyme level in the mitochondria decreased sharply, and therefore the total activity in the 600 g supernatant of the liver homogenate was not much different from the activity in the rats which were not given hemin (Fig. 2) (4). When hemin was injected into rats repeatedly at 2 hr intervals, the enzyme amount in the cytosol fraction increased by more than 5 times as compared to the enzyme level in the control rats, so that the total activity was about 2 times higher in the hemin-injected rats (4). The enzyme accumulating in the liver cytosol fraction after the hemin injection was of the cytosol type, having a larger molecular size (4). Also, the half-life of the cytosol ALA synthetase was elongated more than 5 times when rats received hemin (4).

These observations strongly suggest that hemin inhibits the conversion of the cytosol-type ALA synthetase to the mitochondria-type ALA synthetase of smaller molecular size. The results also suggest that

the induction of ALA synthetase involves two stages
with different susceptibilities to hemin. Namely,
the initial stage of the induction is very sensitive
to hemin and therefore the synthesis of ALA synthetase is strongly suppressed by administration of hemin.
In fact, when hemin was given to normal rats, there
was no accumulation of the enzyme in the cytosol and
the enzyme level in the whole liver decreased markedly
(6). In contrast, once an intensive induction had com-
menced, the synthesis of ALA synthetase becomes considerably resistant to hemin, and under these conditions hemin inhibits the conversion of the cytosol
enzyme to the mitochondrial enzyme.

What might be the mechanism by which the cytosol
ALA synthetase is converted to the mitochondrial ALA
synthetase? Several lines of evidence indicate that
the cytosol ALA synthetase exists in an aggregated
state. For instance, the cytosol ALA synthetase is
converted to a smaller size when treated with high
concentrations of sodium chloride (7,8). In our
case, the apparent molecular weight of ALA synthetase
estimated by gel filtration in the presence of 0.25 M
NaCl was 300,000–350,000, which is approximately half
the size of the original cytosol ALA synthetase. When
this fraction was chromatographed again in the presence of 0.25 M NaCl, sometimes, but not always, the
molecular size became smaller, giving a value of about
120,000–130,000. However, when these fractions were
dialyzed and rechromatographed in the absence of NaCl,
the molecular size returned to the original large size.
These observations suggest that the cytosol ALA synthetase has by nature a tendency to aggregate; for the
conversion of the cytosol ALA synthetase to the mitochondrial ALA synthetase, it seems essential that the
cytosol ALA synthetase is modified in some way so as
to lose the capacity to aggregate.

Considering these possibilities, we tried digestion
of the cytosol enzyme by a snake venom (Naja naja).
The venom treatment caused a considerable decrease of
the enzyme activity. Venom treatment also resulted
in the conversion of the cytosol enzyme to smaller

sizes and the apparent molecular size of the major
fraction obtained after the venom digestion was essentially the same as that of the mitochondrial enzyme.

A hypothetical model for the molecular conversion
of ALA synthetase is presented in Fig. 3. The cytosol
type of ALA synthetase can be dissociated to smaller
aggregates by high concentrations of NaCl; the binding of the ALA synthetase with the unknown cell components (possibly lipoprotein) may also be dissociated
by salts. However, to lose the capacity to aggregate,
the enzyme must be transformed from the soluble form
(designated as S-form) to the mitochondrial form (M-
form), possibly by losing some portion of the enzyme
protein which is responsible to the aggregation. This
step may be catalyzed by a modifying enzyme in the
liver cell, although we have no direct evidence as
yet for the occurrence of the suspected modifying enzyme.

Hoping to find an example which might indicate that
the suspected conversion of the cytosol ALA synthetase
to the mitochondrial enzyme would proceed as a physiological process in the liver, we have examined various
animals and encountered an interesting case with chickens (5). In chicken liver, ALA synthetase increases in
both the cytosol and the mitochondria after the administration of AIA. However, when the enzymes were
examined by gel filtration at different times of induction, the elution pattern of the cytosol ALA synthetase
appeared to exist mainly in relatively smaller molecular forms; but when examined at 8 hr or 12 hr after AIA
enzyme of larger size predominated. These data suggest
that the cytosol ALA synthetase showing a larger molecular size is gradually converted to smaller sizes of
the enzyme in the cytosol and this process of conversion is inhibited by hemin in view of the well-known
fact that heme synthesis in the liver is also increased
in chemically induced porphyria animals.

In the chicken liver the mitochondrial ALA synthetase also exhibited some size heterogeneity and the
elution profile changed according to the duration of
induction (5). When examined at 4 hr, the elution
peak of ALA synthetase corresponded to a molecular

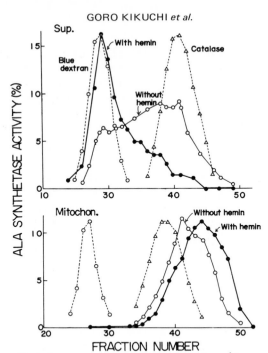

Figure 4: Chickens were given hemin (1 mg/100 g body
weight) at 3 hr after AIA and were killed 1 hr
later. Gel-filtration patterns of ALA synthetases
in the soluble fraction (a) and mitochondria (b)
of chicken liver were examined by using a Sephadex
G-200 column (2.6 x 42 cm) (5). 3 ml fractions
were collected. The activity of ALA synthetase
in each eluate fraction was expressed in terms of
percentage against the total activity recovered.
ALA synthetase was assayed colorimetrically (5).

weight of about 170,000, whereas at 8 hr or 12 hr after AIA, the major peak of ALA synthetase was estimated to have a molecular weight of about 110,000. Apparently the mitochondrial ALA synthetase can exist in two forms and the enzyme with a larger molecular size is gradually converted to a smaller size in mitochondria.

To test the above hypothesis, we performed an experiment shown in Fig. 4. In this experiment, chickens were injected with hemin 3 hr after AIA and sacrificed 1 hr later (4 hr after AIA), then the enzymes were examined by gel filtration. When chickens were given hemin, the majority of the cytosol ALA synthetase was eluted immediately after the void volume. In contrast, in the mitochondria the larger component disappeared and there was a distinct peak of the smaller component (molecular weight of 110,000). It is clear that hemin inhibited the conversion of the larter sized ALA synthetase to a smaller size in the cytosol.

The two forms of ALA synthetase were also found in the liver mitochondria from untreated chickens (5). The molecular conversion of ALA synthetase appears to proceed as a physiological process even in normal animals.

Another important factor which has been shown to markedly affect the induction of ALA synthetase is glucose (9,10). We have observed that the AIA-induced increase of ALA synthetase in both the cytosol and mitochondria was markedly suppressed when glucose was given to rats simultaneously with the administration of AIA; the reduction was particularly significant in the mitochondria. However, when glucose was given to rats 2 hr after AIA, we often noticed that the enzyme level in the cytosol was rather higher than that in the control rats. On the other hand, glucose administration might disturb some hormonal homeostasis. Considering these circumstances, we examined the effects of administration of insulin and cyclic AMP and found that both insulin and cyclic AMP interferred with the conversion of the cytosol ALA synthetase to the mitochondrial ALA synthetase apparently in the

111

same manner as observed with hemin. Namely, when
either insulin or dibutyryl cyclic AMP was given to
rats 2 hr after AIA, the enzyme level in the mitochondria fell sharply and the enzyme level in the
cytosol increased markedly (11). The time courses
of the change of the levels of ALA synthetase in different subcellular fractions after the administration
of insulin or dibutyryl cyclic AMP were quite similar
to those observed after the hemin administration (cf.
Fig. 2). Also the half life of the cytosol enzyme was
elongated by about 3 times when rats were given dibutyryl cyclic AMP. Theophylline mimicked the effect
of cyclic AMP on the induction of ALA synthetase (11).

The present study on the induction and intracellular transfer of ALA synthetase does not provide con-
clusive evidence for the precursor-product relationship between the cytosol ALA synthetase and the mitochondrial ALA synthetase. However, Whiting & Elliot
(8) recently reported that the antibody prepared against
the mitochondrial enzyme from guinea pig liver inhibited the activity of ALA synthetase in the liver
cytosol fraction.

The disaggregation of ALA synthetase seems to be
the most important step in the conversion of the cytosol ALA synthetase to the mitochondrial ALA synthetase.
The molecular conversion appears to involve a proteolytic event, since we have observed that the snake
venom, when heated, failed to convert the larger size
of ALA synthetase to smaller ones. In the chicken
liver the change of the molecular size of ALA synthetase appeared to proceed even in the mitochondria.
Furthermore, ALA synthetase appears to be rapidly degraded in the mitochondria in view of the fact that
the half life of ALA synthetase was very short. The
nature of the intramitochondrial degradation of the
enzyme remains to be clarified.

We have no adequate explanation at present to account for the observation that cyclic AMP exerted
essentially the same effect as that of hemin on the
induction and molecular conversion of ALA synthetase
in the rat liver. The interpretation should be reserved
until the mechanism of the molecular conversion is clarified.

References

1. Granick, S. & Sassa, S. in Metabolic Pathways (H. J. Vogel, ed.), Vol. 5, p. 77, Academic Press, New York (1971).
2. Hayashi, N., Yoda, B. & Kikuchi, G. J. Biochem. 63, 446 (1968).
3. Hayashi, N., Yoda, B. & Kikuchi, G. Arch. Biochem. Biophys. 131, 83 (1969).
4. Hayashi, N., Kurashima, Y. & Kikuchi, G. Arch. Biochem. Biophys. 148, 10 (1972).
5. Ohashi, A. & Kikuchi, G. Arch. Biochem. Biophys. 153, 34 (1972).
6. Ohashi, A. & Sato, S. Tohoku J. Exp. Med. 111, 297 (1973).
7. Scholnick, P. L., Hammaker, L. E. & Marver, H. S. J. Biol. Chem. 247, 4126 (1972).
8. Whiting, M. J. & Elliott, W. H. J. Biol. Chem. 247, 6818 (1972).
9. Tschudy, D. P., Welland, F. H., Collins, A. & Hunter, G., Jr. Metabolism 13, 396 (1963).
10. Marver, H. S., Collins, A., Tschudy, D. P. & Rechcigl, M. J. Biol. Chem. 241, 4323 (1966).
11. Kim, H. J. & Kikuchi, G. J. Biochem. 71, 923 (1972).

δ-AMINOLEVULINIC ACID SYNTHETASE IN MITOCHONDRIA FROM CONTROL AND PORPHYRIC RATS. IDENTICAL PROPERTIES IN PURIFICATION AND RESPONSE TO INTRAMITOCHONDRIAL ENERGY STATE

George M. Patton and Diana S. Beattie

Department of Biochemistry
Mount Sinai School of Medicine
of the City University of New York

The initial step in the biosynthesis of heme in mammalian liver cells involves the mitochondrial enzyme δ-aminolevulinic acid (ALA) synthetase (1). This enzyme, which catalyzes the proposed rate-limiting step in the over-all heme biosynthetic sequence, is induced by a variety of chemicals which also cause an experimental porphyria (2-5). The increase in ALA synthetase activity after administration of porphyrogenic drugs requires protein synthesis (4), and this elevated enzymatic activity decays rapidly with a half-life of about 1 hr. when inhibitors of protein synthesis are administered (6,7). A recent report from this laboratory, however, indicated that the maximum activity of ALA synthetase, assayed in dilute sonicated mitochondria, was identical in both control and porphyric rats (8). These results imply the existence of a specific labile regulatory protein, or proteins, which act to increase the activity, but not the actual amount of ALA synthetase in the mitochondria. In the present study, several physical and regulatory properties of ALA synthetase in mitochondria from both control and porphyric rats were examined in an attempt to elucidate the mechanism of the increase in activity. No significant differences were

115

observed in the properties of ALA synthetase from either control or porphyric rats. Furthermore, the response of the enzyme to changes in the energy charge or the redox state of the mitochondria was identical in both types of mitochondria.

Materials and Methods

Rats weighing 75-100 g were fasted for 8 hr. and injected with 25 mg/100 g body weight of 3,5-dicarbethoxy-1,4-dihydrocollidine (DDC) and continued fasting until sacrifice 17 hrs. later. Livers were removed and mitochondria were prepared according to the method of Beattie et al. (9) in 0.25M sucrose containing 0.01M Tris, pH 7.6, and 0.001M EDTA. Mitochondria were suspended in the isolation medium at a concentration of 1 mg/ml and sonicated for 10 sec. at full power with a model W1850 Bronson Sonifier.

Mitochondria were fractionated by the digitonin-Lubrol method of Schnaitman & Greenawalt (10). The lubrol soluble (matrix) fraction was further centrifuged at 165,000 x g for 120 min. ALA synthetase was assayed as previously described (8) in 2 ml of a potassium-free incubation mixture containing 100 mM glycine, 50 mM Tris (pH 7.3), 20 mM $MgCl_2$, 10 mM EDTA, 0.1 mM pyridoxal phosphate and 1 μCi of either [^{14}C] succinate or [^{14}C]-glutamate. With sonicated mitochondria, 1 mM ATP, 100 μM reduced Coenzyme A and 250 μg of Succinyl-CoA synthetase (prepared by the method of Lasceles [11] from R. Spheroides) were also added. ALA was determined by the method of Ebert et al. (12).

[2,3-^{14}C] Succinate (22 mCi/mMol) and uniformly labeled [^{14}C] L-glutamate (10 mCi/mMole) were obtained from Amersham-Searle. Digitonin was obtained from Sigma and recrystallized from ethanol and DDC from Eastman. Protein was determined by the method of Lowry et al. (13) with bovine serum albumin as standard.

TABLE I

Effect of Succinate Concentration on ALA Synthetase Activity in Sonicated Mitochondria.

Succinate	Control 100µg	500µg	Porphyric 100µg	500µg Protein
	nmoles/mg protein			
5 mM	1.2	1.51	3.3	1.4
1 mM	0.92	0.95	0.94	0.83
0.25 mM	0.85	0.77	1.03	0.65
0.05 mM	1.0	0.62	1.05	0.57

TABLE II

Partial Purification of ALA Synthetase

	C O N T R O L		P O R P H Y R I C	
	Specific Activity	Total Activity	Specific Activity	Total Activity
	cpm/mg	cpm	cpm/mg	cpm
Intact Mitochondria	1060	–	12,600	–
Sonicated Mitochondria	10,400	14.4×10^5	20,300	19.9×10^5
Inner Membrane	9,230	9.4×10^5	20,000	16.6×10^5
Lubrol Supernatant	25,600	5.1×10^5	73,300	11.0×10^5

Results and Discussion

We have previously demonstrated (8) that no increase in ALA synthetase activity occurs during porphyria when the enzyme is assayed under optimal conditions with dilute suspensions of sonicated mitochondria as a source of enzyme and $[^{14}C]$succinate as
substrate. Activity was linear with both time and
protein concentrations and independent of substrate
concentration. Since these assays were performed with
very dilute protein suspensions (100 µg of sonicated
mitochondria) and low concentrations of substrate
(0.05 - 0.2 mM succinate), we have reinvestigated
the effect of succinate over a wider concentration
range (0.05 - 5.0 mM) and at higher protein concentrations (100 µg and 500 µg of sonicated mitochondrial
protein). As seen in Table I, the specific activity
of ALA synthetase in sonicated mitochondria obtained
from both control and porphyric rats is identical.
The activity remains constant over the entire range
of succinate concentrations tested; and furthermore,
had the same activity on a per mg of protein basis
when either 100 µg or 500 µg of sonicated mitochondria
were present. The values obtained with 5 mM succinate
are subject to considerable variation as very low
counts are obtained when 1 µCi of $[^{14}C]$ succinate is
diluted with such a large amount of unlabeled succinate. Several groups have observed that the increase
in ALA synthetase activity during experimental porphyria is prevented by inhibitors of cytoplasmic RNA
and protein synthesis (6,7). However, the results
of our previous studies (8) have suggested that the
actual amount of ALA synthetase may not vary in control and porphyric rats. These observations imply
that some specific product or products of cytoplasmic
protein synthesis are capable of altering the activity
of ALA synthetase in intact mitochondria. Attempts to
demonstrate such an activation by incubating mitochondria obtained from control rats with various cell
fractions obtained from porphyric rats, or to demonstrate the reverse process using mitochondria obtained

from porphyric rats and various fractions from control
rats have been singularly unsuccessful.

We have next attempted to determine whether the
activation of ALA synthetase in intact mitochondria
causes any gross changes in the physical properties
of the enzyme. Therefore, ALA synthetase was partially purified from mitochondria obtained from both
control and porphyric rats (Table II). The enzymatic
activity of intact mitochondria from the porphyric
rats is nearly 12-fold greater than the activity of
intact mitochondria obtained from control rats. In
the sonicated mitochondria, the specific activity of
the enzyme from porphyric rats is 2-fold greater than
that from control rats. In this particular experiment,
the specific activity of the enzyme in sonicated mitochondria from control rats is lower than usual. The
specific activity of ALA synthetase in sonicated mitochondria from both porphyric and control rats varies
from animal to animal in the range of 10,000-25,000
cpm/mg.

When the mitochondria from both control and porphyric rats are fractionated into inner and outer membrane fractions, all the detectable enzymatic activity
is present in the inner membrane. After treatment of
the inner membrane with Lubrol (1 mg/10 mg protein)
all of the detectable activity is solubilized. Approximately 80% of ALA synthetase activity does not precipitate when the Lubrol-treated inner membrane is centrifuged at 165,000 x g for 2 hr. (Lubrol Sup.). The
enzyme from both sources required dithioerythritol
for maximum stability, showed similar sensitivity to
various salts and had the same apparent molecular
weight after chromatography on Sephadex G-200 (running
just behind the peak at the void volume).

We have previously reported that the activity of
ALA synthetase in intact mitochondria is increased 4-
fold by acute ethanol intoxication (14). Ethanol is
unique among inducers of ALA synthetase in that the
metabolism and metabolic consequences of ethanol intoxication are well-characterized. Since ethanol is
known to alter the intracellular redox state (15) and

TABLE III

Effect of Respiratory Inhibitors and Uncouplers on ALA Synthetase Activity
in Intact Mitochondria

	C O N T R O L	P O R P H Y R I C
Additions	% Control [Range]	% Control
+ Rotenone (6)	-61% [46% - 77%]	-63%
+ Valinomycin (5)	+51% [20% - 110%]	+64%
+ Dinitrophenol (5)	+70% [40% - 110%]	+90%
+ Oligomycin (4)	-10% [0 - 20%]	No effect
	Control value = 720 cpm/mg	Porphyric value = 3800 cpm/mg

Numbers in parenthesis indicate number of experiments.

TABLE IV

Effect of Changing NADH/NAD$^+$ and ATP/ADP Ratios on ALA Synthetase
Activity in Intact Mitochondria

Additions	S U C C I N A T E		G L U T A M A T E	
	Control	Porphyric	Control	Porphyric
		cpm/mg		
None	610	3900	886	1870
Oligo, DNP, ADP	540	3800	1886	1980
Oligo, DNP, ATP	610	5280	1090	3090
Oligo, rot, ADP	90	430	795	745
Oligo, rot, ATP	180	760	840	1050

Oligo= oligomycin, Rot= rotenone, DNP= dinitrophenol

thereby affect the regulation of energy metabolism, we examined the effects of various respiratory inhibitors to see if the redox state [(NAD$^+$)/(NADH)ratio] or phosphate potential [(ATP)/(ADP)(Pi)] had any effect on the activity of ALA synthetase in intact mitochondria (Table III). Rotenone, a respiratory inhibitor which causes an accumulation of NADH by blocking its oxidation by the respiratory chain, severely inhibited ALA synthetase activity. Both valinomycin, a potassium specific ionophore which allows potassium to equilibrate across the mitochondrial membrane in response to a charge gradient, and carbonyl cyanide m-chlorophenyl hydrazone (CCP) or 2,4 dinitrophenol (DNP), classical uncouplers of oxidative phosphorylation, significantly stimulated ALA synthetase activity. The action of all of these compounds results in lower levels of both ATP and NADH. Oligomycin which blocks ATP synthesis without uncoupling respiration, thus leading to lower ATP and higher NADH levels, had no effect on enzymatic activity. Mitochondria from both control and porphyric rats responded identically to the inhibitors when succinate was used as substrate. Similar experiments using α-ketoglutarate or glutamate as substrate yielded appreciably identical results.

Next, an attempt was made to regulate the NAD$^+$/NADH and ATP/ADP ratios simultaneously to learn what effect these ratios had on ALA synthetase activity (Table IV). Oligomycin was added to control the ATP/ADP ratio independently of NAD$^+$/NADH ratio which was varied by adding an uncoupler, to cause low NADH levels, or the respiratory inhibitor, rotenone, to cause high NADH levels. As the mitochondrial membrane is impermeable to pyridine nucleotides and as adenine nucleotides are transported across the mitochondrial membrane by an exchange carrier mechanism (16), the intramitochondrial levels of the pairs NAD$^+$/NADH and ATP/ADP should remain constant. As seen in Table IV, ALA synthetase activity in intact mitochondria obtained from both control and porphyric rats is increased by high ATP levels and decreased by high NADH levels when either succinate or glutamate was the substrate. It should be noted that none of the inhibitors tested had any effect on the activity of ALA synthetase in sonicated mitochondria. Furthermore, addition of calcium, an ion which is actively accumulated and extruded by mitochondria, had no effect on ALA synthetase activity in intact mitochondria.

Although ALA synthetase activity can be varied by changing the intramitochondrial, ATP/ADP or NAD$^+$/NADH ratios, these changes do not appear to be responsible for the increase in ALA synthetase activity in experimental porphyria. Different manipulations do cause changes in enzymatic activity over a 4-5 fold range; however, the maximum activity obtained is at most two times the control values. This increase is well below the 10-20 fold increase in enzymatic activity observed in mitochondria obtained from rats made porphyric by treatment with DDC. The observation that ALA synthetase activity in mitochondria from both control and porphyric rats respond in an identical fashion to the energy state of the mitochondria, also indicates that these changes are not responsible for the increased activity in the porphyric animal. These results, however, do tend to support the concept that ALA synthetase of both control and porphyric eats is the same enzymatic protein. The enzyme from both types of mitochondria purifies in the same way and also responds identically to changes in both the redox state and the energy charge of the mitochondria. Hence, whatever is responsible for the increase in ALA synthetase activity of the enzyme is controlled by the metabolic state of the mitochondria.

Acknowledgements

Supported in part by Grant HD04007 from the United States Public Health Service.

References

1. Granick, S. & Sassa, S. in "Metabolic Pathways" (H. J. Vogel, ed.), Vol. 5, 3rd Ed. pp. 79-141, Academic Press, New York (1971).

2. Granick, S. & Urata, G. J. Biol. Chem. 238, 821 (1963).
3. Tschudy, D. P., Welland, F. H., Collins, A., & Hunter, G., Jr. Metabolism 13, 396 (1964).
4. Granick, S. J. Biol. Chem. 241, 1359 (1966).
5. Marver, H. S., Collins, A., Tschudy, D. P., & Rechcigl, M., Jr. J. Biol. Chem. 241, 4323 (1966).
6. Tschudy, D. P., Marver, H. S. & Collins, A. Biochem. Biophys. Res. Commun. 21, 480 (1965).
7. Hayashi, N., Yoda, B. & Kikuchi, G. Arch. Biochem. Biophys. 131, 83 (1969).
8. Patton, G. M. & Beattie, D. S. J. Biol. Chem. 248, 4467 (1973).
9. Beattie, D. S., Basford, R. E. & Koritz, S. B. J. Biol. Chem. 242, 3366 (1967).
10. Schnaitman, C. & Greenawalt, J. W. J. Cell Biol. 38, 158 (1968).
11. Lascelles, J. Biochem. J. 72, 508, 1959.
12. Ebert, P. S., Tschudy, D. P., Choudhry, J. N., & Chirigos, M. A. Biochim. Biophys. Acta 208, 236 (1970).
13. Lowry, O. H., Rosebrough, N. J., Farr, A. L. & Randall, R. J. J. Biol. Chem. 193, 265 (1951).
14. Beattie, D. S., Patton, G. M. & Rubin, E. Enzyme, in press.
15. Leiber, C. S. Adv. Internal Med. 14, 151 (1968).
16. Klingenberg, M. Essays in Biochemistry 6, 119 (1970).

REGULATION OF THE ACETYL COENZYME A CARBOXYLASE CONTENT OF MAMMALIAN AND AVIAN LIVER

Shosaku Numa, Kaoru Kitajima, Hirobumi Teraoka and Shigetada Nakanishi

Department of Medical Chemistry
Kyoto University Faculty of Medicine
Kyoto, Japan

Acetyl coenzyme A carboxylase (acetyl-CoA:carbon dioxide ligase (ADP), EC 6.4.1.2), which catalyzes the formation of malonyl-CoA from acetyl-CoA, plays a critical role in the regulation of long-chain fatty acid biosynthesis (1,2). The level of activity of this enzyme in liver fluctuates in accord with the rate of fatty acid synthesis under different dietary, hormonal, developmental and genetic conditions of the aminal (1,2). In the present work, we investigated the questions, whether these fluctuations in the level of acetyl-CoA carboxylase activity are actually due to changes in the quantity of the enzyme protein, and if so, whether these changes are ascribed to variations in the rate of enzyme synthesis or in that of enzyme degradation. For this purpose, we used animals in various metabolic states associated with elevated or depressed fatty acid synthesis. Furthermore, an attempt was made with the use of cultured liver cells to search for the factors that are directly responsible for determining the acetyl-CoA carboxylase content of the liver.

Studies with Animals

The animals studied were as shown in Table I. Immunochemical titrations of liver extracts derived from animals in various states demonstrated that the changes in the level of acetyl–CoA carboxylase activity are accompanied by proportionate changes in the quantity of immunochemically reactive protein. For these experiments, we used antibody prepared by injecting rabbits with homogeneous rat (3) or chicken liver acetyl–CoA carboxylase (5); the antibody against the rat liver enzyme was found to cross–react with the mouse liver enzyme. In addition, Ouchterlony double diffusion analyses with enzyme preparations obtained from rats and mice in different states showed the completeness of connections of the precipitation bands, indicating that carboxylase molecules are immunologically similar in all the states. Furthermore, enzyme preparations derived from genetically obese mice (C57BL/6J–ob) and from normal mice exhibited no qualitative differences with respect to kinetic properties and heat stability. All these results indicate that the wide variations in the level of acetyl–CoA carboxylase activity in liver extracts observed under various conditions are actually due to changes in the quantity of the enzyme.

The tissue content of an enzyme is generally determined by a balance between the rate of synthesis and the rate of degradation of the enzyme. Under steady-state conditions, the enzyme content is related to these rates as follows:

$$E = k_S/k_d \qquad (1)$$

where E is the enzyme content per mass, k_S is a zero-order rate constant of synthesis per mass, and k_d is a first–order rate constant of degradation expressed as reciprocal of time (6). We therefore investigated whether the above–mentioned fluctuations in the acetyl–CoA carboxylase content of the liver are due to changes in the rate of enzyme synthesis or in that of enzyme degradation. The rate of carboxylase synthesis was assessed by injecting animals intraperitoneally with a dose of (^{3}H)leucine and shortly thereafter determining the incorporation of isotopic leucine into the enzyme, which was isolated from the soluble supernatant by immunoprecipitation with specific antibody. Since

TABLE I.

Synthesis and Degradation of Hepatic Acetyl-CoA Carboxylase
Under Various Conditions*

Animals	Conditions	Enzyme content**	Rate of synthesis**	Rate constant of degradation	Half-life	k_s/k_d
		(E)	(k_s)	(k_d)	(hr)	
Rats	Normal	1	1	1	59	1
	Fasted for 48 hr.	0.28	0.59	1.90	31	0.31
	Fasted for 48 hr and subsequently refed a fat-free diet for 72 hr.	3.76	4.05	1.07	55	3.78
	Alloxan-diabetic	0.53	0.54	1.00	59	0.54
Mice	Normal	1	1	1	67	1
	Genetically obese	10.2 (3.54)	7.75 (2.69)	0.58	115	13.4 (4.64)
Chicks	2-day-old	1	1	Turnover not detectable		
	10-day old	54.2 (15.3)	18.3 (5.14)		46	

* E, k_s, k_d and k_s/k_d are given as values relative to those under certain standard conditions. Data for rats and mice were taken from Nakanishi and Numa (3,4).

** Per liver except for figures in parentheses, which represent values per unit weight of liver.

the extent of labeling of the carboxylase depends on
that of total soluble liver protein, the synthesis
rate of the carboxylase relative to that of total protein was calculated by dividing the radioactivity incorporated into the enzyme by that incorporated into
total protein. The rate of carboxylase degradation
was measured by following the time course of loss of
isotope from prelabeled enzyme. The decay of radioactivity in the enzyme was found to follow first-order
kinetics. The results of these measurements are summarized in Table I. It is evident from this table
that the increase or decrease in the carboxylase content in fat-free refed or alloxan-diabetic rats can
be attributed to accelerated or retarded synthesis of
the enzyme, while the rate constant of carboxylase
degradation is essentially the same in normally fed,
fat-free refed and alloxan-diabetic rats. On the
other hand, the decrease in the carboxylase content in
fasted rats is effected both by retarded synthesis and
by accelerated breakdown. The elevated carboxylase
content in genetically obese mice is due mainly to a
rise in the rate of synthesis, and in a minor degree,
to a decrease in the rate constant of degradation.
The large increase in the carboxylase content during
growth of chicks following hatching – which can be
regarded as an adaptive response to the change from
high-fat nutrition to high-carbohydrate nutrition
upon hatching – is ascribed to a marked elevation of
the rate of synthesis. It is noteworthy that the
degradation of hepatic acetyl-CoA carboxylase in 2-
day-old chicks was too slow to be detectable. An
unusually slow degradation rate was reported also for
malic enzyme, another lipogenic enzyme, in the liver
of neonatal chicks (7). The results obtained with
normally fed and fasted rats are in general agreement
with those of Majerus & Kilburn (8), although these
investigators found slightly shorter values for the
half-life of the carboxylase (50 and 18 hours respectively for normally fed and fasted rats).

In the experiments to determine the rate of degradation, reutilization of (^{3}H)leucine may lead to an

overestimation of the half-life (9). However, this
does not appear to be of major significance in our
experiments except for growing chicks; the half-life
for degradation of total soluble liver protein, estimated simultaneously by means of this isotope, was 91,
70, 89 and 82 hours in normally fed, fasted, fat-free
refed and alloxan-diabetic rats, 109 and 124 hours in
normal and obese mice, respectively. In 10-day old
chicks, the half-life for breakdown of total soluble
liver protein was 72 hours, while no measurable turnover was observed in 2-day old chicks.

The results given in Table I reveal that the variations in the content of hepatic acetyl-CoA carboxylase
can always be accounted for at least in part by changes
in the rate of enzyme synthesis. In most cases, the
carboxylase content is determined exclusively or principally by an altered synthesis rate. The only instance
in which a change in the rate constant of degradation
plays an important regulatory role is the state of
starvation. In fasted animals, not only hepatic acetyl-
CoA carboxylase but also fatty acid synthetase (10,11)
and malic enzyme (7), which are also involved in lipo-
genesis, are degraded more rapidly than in fed animals.
The decrease in the content of these enzymes upon starvation is due both to retarded synthesis and to accelerated breakdown. Fasted animals are not in a steady
state, while the other animals studied, except growing
chicks, can be assumed to be in steady states. Thus,
it is suggested that control of the rate of enzyme
degradation makes a significant contribution to the
regulation of enzyme content only when the animal
deviates from a steady state to get adjusted to a new
environment. This concept is supported also by the
finding of Schimke (12) on rat liver arginase. In
fat-free refed and alloxan-diabetic rats as well as
in obese mice, the values for the carboxylase content
predicted from the ratio k_s/k_d according to Equation
(1) agree fairly well with the values actually found.

Studies with Cultured Liver Cells

The next question is which factors are directly
responsible for determining the content of hepatic

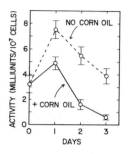

Figure 1: Effect of corn oil on the level of acetyl-
CoA carboxylase activity in cultured liver cells.
JTC-25·P3 cells grown to confluence were incubated
in the medium DM-120 (14) in the presence and absence of approximately 0.1 mM corn oil (concentration as oleo-dilinolein). Corn oil was added in
the form of its albumin complex, which was prepared
by sonicating a mixture containing corn oil and
fatty acid-free bovine serum albumin in the molar
ratio 10:1. Cultures without corn oil received
fatty acid-free bovine serum albumin at the corresponding concentration. At the times indicated,
cells were harvested, and the activity of acetyl-
CoA carboxylase was assayed at 37°C by the (^{14}C)
bicarbonate-fixation method as described previously
(3). Results are given as means ± S.E. for three
experiments.

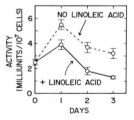

Figure 2: Effect of linoleic acid on the level of
acetyl-CoA carboxylase activity in cultured liver
cells. Experimental details were the same as described for Fig. 1 escept that approximately 0.01 mM
linoleic acid as its albumin complex was added to
cultures when indicated. The fatty acid-albumin
Complex was prepared by the method of Spector &
Hoak (17).

acetyl–CoA carboxylase through changes in the rates
of its synthesis and degradation. In order to investi-
gate this problem, we used cultured liver cells JTC-
25·P3 (13), which were derived from rat liver cells.
These cells can be grown in a protein- and lipid-free
synthetic medium, thus allowing one to avoid the complex physiological interactions encountered in whole
animals. In the experiment shown in Figure 1, we
examined the effect of corn oil added to the medium
on the level of acetyl–CoA carboxylase activity in cultured liver cells. The activity level fluctuated periodically with changes of the medium. It attained a
maximal level one day after the medium was changed,
and fell gradually thereafter. When cells were cultured in the presence of corn oil, the level of carboxylase activity was reduced markedly as compared
with that in control cells. Corn oil was added in
the form of its complex with bovine serum albumin,
but albumin itself had practically no effect on the
activity level. Neither the growth (tested by the
simplified replicate culture method [15]) nor the
viability (tested by erythrosin B exclusion [16]) of
the cells were affected appreciably by the addition
of corn oil. The action of corn oil depended on its
concentration in the medium; the activity level decreased with increasing oil concentration.

The fatty acids that occur most frequently in corn
oil are linoleic acid and oleic acid. Figure 2 com-
pares the levels of acetyl–CoA carboxylase activity
in liver cells cultured in the presence and absence
of linoleic acid. The addition of linoleic acid
clearly depressed the activity level despite the fact
that the fatty acid hardly affected the growth and
viability of the cells. Oleic acid was likewise shown
to have a similar dampening effect on the carboxylase.

Furthermore, immunochemical titrations revealed
that the decrease in the level of acetyl–CoA carboxylase activity observed upon addition of linoleic acid
or oleic acid is actually due to a corresponding reduction of the enzyme content of cultured liver cells.
For this experiment, antibody prepared against homogeneous rat liver acetyl–CoA carboxylase was utilized,

131

since it was found to cross-react with the carboxylase from JTC-25·P3 cells.

Analogous dampening effects of fatty acids on the acetyl-CoA carboxylase content were demonstrated also in human skin fibroblasts (18) as well as in yeast (19). All these results suggest that fatty acids or compounds metabolically related to them may be involved in the repression of acetyl-CoA carboxylase.

Summary

The content of hepatic acetyl Coenzyme A carboxylase, which plays a critical role in the control of fatty acid biosynthesis, is regulated mainly by changes in the rate of enzyme synthesis rather than by changes in the rate of enzyme degradation. In the state of starvation, however, accelerated degradation of the enzyme also plays an important regulatory role. Fatty acids or compounds metabolically related to them may be involved in the repression of the carboxylase.

Acknowledgements

The authors are indebted to Dr. H. Katsuta for kindly providing JTC-25·P3 cells. This work was supported in part by research grants from the Ministry of Education of Japan, the Toray Science Foundation, the Japanese Foundation of Metabolism and Diseases, the Japan Waksman Foundation, the Iyakushigen Foundation, the Naito Foundation, the Tanabe Amino Acid Research Foundation and the Japanese Medical Association.

References

1. Numa, S., Nakanishi, S., Hashimoto, T., Iritani, N. & Okazaki, T. Vitamins and Hormones 28, 213 (1970).
2. Numa, S. Ergebnisse der Physiologie 69, 53 (1974).
3. Nakanishi, S. & Numa, S. Eur. J. Biochem. 16, 161 (1970).

4. Nakanishi, S. & Numa, S.   Proc. Nat. Acad. Sci. USA 68, 2288 (1971).
5. Numa, S.   Methods in Enzymology 14, 9 (1969).
6. Schimke, R. T. & Doyle, D.   Annual Rev. Biochem. 39, 929 (1970).
7. Silpananta, P. & Goodridge, A. G.   J. Biol. Chem. 246, 5754 (1971).
8. Majerus, P. W. & Kilburn, E.   J. Biol. Chem. 244, 6254 (1971).
9. Koch, B. L.   J. Theor. Biol. 3, 283 (1962).
10. Tweto, J. & Larrabee, A. R.   J. Biol. Chem. 247, 4900 (1972).
11. Volpe, J. J., Lyles, T. O., Roncari, D. A. K., & Vagelos, P. R.   J. Biol. Chem. 248, 2502 (1973).
12. Schimke, R. T.   J. Biol. Chem. 239, 3808 (1964).
13. Katsuta, H. & Takaoka, T.   Methods in Cell Biology 6, 1 (1973).
14. Katsuta, H., Takaoka, T. & Kikuchi, K.   Japan. J. Exp. Med. 31, 125 (1961).
15. Katsuta, H., Takaoka, T., Oishi, Y., Baba, T. & Chang, K. C.   Japan, J. Exp. Med. 24, 125 (1954).
16. Phillips, H. J. & Terryberry, J. E.   Exp. Cell Res. 13, 341 (1957).
17. Spector, A. A. & Hoak, J. C.   Anal. Biochem. 32, 297 (1969).
18. Jacobs, R. A., Sly, W. S. & Majerus, P. W.   J. Biol. Chem. 248, 1268 (1973).
19. Kamiryo, T. & Numa, S.   FEBS Letters 38, 29 (1973).

133

PROTEIN TURNOVER DURING DEVELOPMENT

Paul J. Fritz, E. Lucile White, and Juraj Osterman

Department of Pharmacology
Pennsylvania State University College of Medicine
Hershey, Pennsylvania 17033

Kenneth M. Pruitt

Laboratory of Molecular Biology
University of Alabama in Birmingham
Birmingham, Alabama 35233

Protein turnover in the tissues of mature animals has been extensively studied during recent years (1,2). There have also been many reports describing variations in protein levels in animal tissues during growth and development (3). Furthermore, in several instances, rates of synthesis and the turnover of particular enzymes have been estimated during growth and development (4-7). However, the roles of the rates of synthesis and degradation in regulating protein levels during development have received little attention. The purpose of this report is to discuss the influence of these rates on protein levels in terms of a model that is applicable to tissues at any stage of their development.

Most workers agree with Zilversmit (8-9) who originally proposed that turnover, as applicable to biochemistry, be defined as the rate of renewal or the rate of replacement of a specified substance. While we have no basic disagreement with this definition, we feel, along with Reiner (10), that the definition need not be limited to the steady state condition, as

specified by Zilversmit, but should be extended to
situations, such as development, where the protein
levels may be changing significantly over a given
period of time. Proteins are being made and broken
down when their levels are changing as well as when
they are constant. The level may either increase,
decrease, or remain the same, but regardless of the
direction of change, replacement, or turnover, is
still going on during a given time interval. When
there is a net accumulation of a protein in a given
tissue, the rate of synthesis is greater than the
rate of degradation. Here the protein is being replaced at a rate equal to the rate of degradation.
If there is a net increase in the tissue level of a
particular protein, then the degradation rate exceeds
the synthesis rate and the rate of replacement (turnover) must equal the rate of synthesis. Thus, in a
situation other than steady state, turnover is represented by the rate of synthesis or the rate of degradation, <u>whichever is smaller</u>.

We have reported on changes in pyruvate kinase
levels in rat tissues during development (11) and
would now like to address ourselves to the question
of how these changes are determined. The first step
is to sort out the contribution of rates of synthesis
and degradation, since if the enzyme level changes,
these two rates are unequal. To analyze the protein
level versus time data we have devised a kinetic
method that takes into account the potential variability of the rates of synthesis and degradation.
The basic equation is:

$$\frac{dP}{dt} = S(t) - L(t)P. \qquad (1)$$

This equation expresses the total rate of change in
the amount of tissue protein, P, in terms of the time,
t, and the time dependent functions $S(t)$ and $L(t)$.
$S(t)$ includes the contribution of all processes which
increase the amount of P, while $L(t)$ includes the contribution of all processes which effectively remove P
from the tissue. The value of both functions must be
either positive or zero. The equation assumes only

that the output, $L(t)P$, is at least first order with
respect to the level of protein under investigation.
Regulatory events within the cell alter protein levels
by producing biochemical changes which alter the values
of the input and output functions $S(t)$ and $L(t)$.   In
order to evaluate these functions by utilizing equation 1, at least two sets of data or assumptions are
required. If P is known as a function of t, then it
is necessary either to have experimental values for
$S(t)$ or $L(t)$ or to make assumptions regarding them.
In the absence of experimentally determined values,
we have used assumed specific forms for these functions in order to estimate how changes in rates of
synthesis and degradation could account for changes
in the pyruvate kinase levels measured in three rat
tissues during development. The forms we used are sums
of inverse exponentials because these forms have the
mathematical property of reaching a constant value as
time increases, but allow for changes in the rates
during the time before steady state is reached. The
choice of this particular form for the functions is
not mathematically unique. In any particular case,
other types of functions might work as well or better.
However, the inverse exponentials have the advantages
of generality (they can be used to represent any mathematically well-behaved function) and convenience for
computer analysis. Although the parameters have no
distinct relationship to specific molecular events,
this method of analysis still has utility in sorting
out the net contributions of variations in $S(t)$ and
$L(t)$ to changes in protein level.

    After substituting the inverse exponential func-
tions, equation 1 becomes:

$$\frac{dP}{dt} = S(\infty) + \Sigma s_i e^{-\sigma_i t} - \{L(\infty) + \Sigma l_i e^{-\lambda_i t}\}P, \qquad (2)$$

where P = the protein level at time t and the two sets
of numbers $\{s_i, \sigma_i\}$ and $\{l_i, \lambda_i\}$, are constants which
characterize the time dependence of the input and out-
put functions, respectively, for a given protein. Individual values of s_i and l_i may be positive or

137

negative but σ_i and λ_i must be positive. $S(\infty)$ and $L(\infty)$ are positive constants which are the limiting values of the input and output functions at large t. As the steady state level is approached, the exponential terms in equation 2 become negligible and the equation approaches:

$$\frac{dP}{dt} = S(\infty) - L(\infty)P. \tag{3}$$

When the steady state level $P(\infty)$ has been reached, the rate of change is zero and we can write:

$$P(\infty) = \frac{S(\infty)}{L(\infty)} \tag{4}$$

Therefore, since $S(\infty)$ and $L(\infty)$ are constants, equation 3 is identical in form to the simple zero order–first order rate equation used extensively in studies of mature animal tissue proteins (1).

Estimates of the rates of synthesis and degradation of pyruvate kinase during development using the protein level versus time data and equation 2 were obtained by the following procedure:

(a) The measured values of pyruvate kinase at the various times during development were fitted to the following equation:

$$P = P(\infty) + \Sigma b_i e^{-\beta_i t} \tag{5}$$

The set of constants b_i, β_i were determined by non-linear least squares analysis.

(b) The equation obtained in (a) was differentiated to obtain a set of dP/dt values for the P versus t curve.

(c) The dP/dt values obtained in (b) were used together with their corresponding P's and equation 2 in order to obtain S(t) and L(t). The coefficients and exponents in equation 2 were obtained by non-linear least squares analysis.

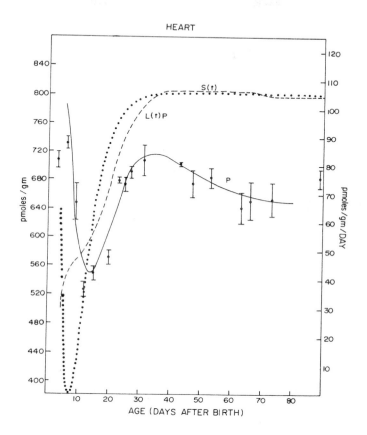

Figure 1. Developmental changes in rat heart pyruvate kinase. The data are means (closed circles) ± 1 standard error of 4 to 8 animals. The dotted line labeled S(t) and the dashed line labeled L(t)P represent the estimated values for the rates (pmoles/gm/day) of input and output, respectively. The curve labeled P (pmoles/gm) was obtained by numerical integration of equation 2.

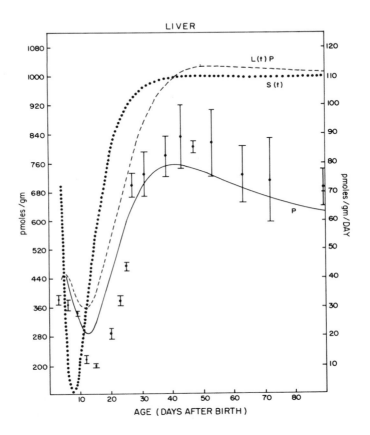

Figure 2. Developmental changes in rat liver pyruvate kinase. For details see legend to figure 1.

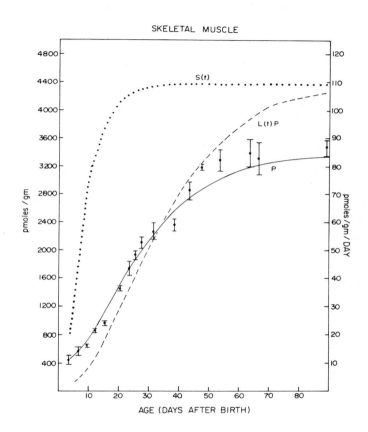

Figure 3. Developmental changes in rat skeletal muscle pyruvate kinase. For details see legend to figure 1.

The results of the analysis are shown in Figs. 1, 2 and 3 for pyruvate kinase from rat heart, liver and skeletal muscle, respectively. There are several permutations of the rate of synthesis and rate of degradation parameters that could account for changes in protein levels over a given period of time. Among the less intuitively obvious that are represented in the figures are (a) the protein level decreases while the rate of synthesis increases (heart and liver around ten days after birth) (b) the protein level increases while the rate of synthesis is constant (liver around 35 days after birth) (c) the protein level decreases while the rate of synthesis is constant (liver from 40 to 80 days after birth). The primary consideration and the explanation for all these observations is that when the rates of synthesis and degradation are unequal the protein level must change. Whether the level increases or decreases is determined by which is greater, the rate of synthesis or the rate of degradation. We would also like to emphasize that the <u>rate at which the enzyme level changes is determined solely by the magnitude of the difference between the rates of synthesis and degradation.</u>

It is clear from equation 1 that the change in the level of P over any time period is determined by summing the amount of the new protein put into the system during that period and subtracting the amount of protein taken out of the system during that same period. Another way of expressing this is that the magnitude of the change in protein levels is determined by the magnitude of the difference between the area under the curves representing the rates of synthesis and degradation for that time period. It follows that the level of P at any time would be determined by adding the value arrived at in this manner to the value of P at the beginning of the time period. This is true for all times during development including the steady state. Although it is correct, as seen from equation 4, that for particular values of $L(\infty)$ and $S(\infty)$ there is only one possible steady state level of P, the differences in steady state levels of

TABLE I.

Pyruvate Kinase Turnover in Rat Tissues

Tissue	Steady state level picomoles/g	k_s pm/g/day	k_d day^{-1}	Half-life days
Liver	550	110	0.200	3.5
Heart	644	106	0.164	4.2
Skeletal Muscle	3,362	108	0.032	21.6

TABLE II.

Turnover Data for Several Rat Liver Enzymes[a]

Enzyme	picomoles/ liver	units/g liver	picomoles/ unit	Molecular weight	k_d day^{-1}	k_s pm/g/day	$t_{1/2}$ (hours)	Ref.
Tyrosine amino transferase	3,000	1.8	1,670	115,000	11	33,000	1.5	12,13
Serine dehydratase	594	4.4	135	64,000	3.20	1,900	5.2	14,15,16
Acetyl CoA Carboxylase	89	.28	318	409,000	.277	24.6	59	17
Aldolase	26,250	10.5	2,500	160,000	.248	6,500	67.2	18
Glyceraldehyde phosphate dehydrogenase	3,500	49	71.5	140,000	.224	784	74.4	18
Pyruvate kinase-1	550	23.4	23.5	208,000	.200	110	84	11
δ-Aminolevulinate dehydratase [b]	1,330	.05	26,600	250,000	.138	183	120	19,20
Lactate dehydrogenase-5	2,199	176	12.5	140,000	.036	79.2	462	21

[a] To illustrate how the values in this table were calculated from information in the literature, the following sample calculation for rat liver serine dehydratase is presented. Information (A) given: Molecular weight-64,000 (Nakagawa and Kimura, 1969); Specific activity of purified enzyme-115 international units per mg of protein (Nakagawa et al., 1967); Steady state enzyme level (uninduced)-4.4 international units per gram of liver (Jost et al., 1968); Half life-5.2 hours (Jost et al., 1968).
(B) Calculated:
    (i) 1 mg serine dehydratase ÷ 6.4 x 10^4 mg/mmole = 15.6 x 10^3 pmole
   (ii) 15.6 x 10^3 pmole ÷ 115 units = 135 pmole/unit
  (iii) 4.4 units/g liver x 135 pmole/unit = 594 pmole/g liver
   (iv) $t_{1/2}$ = 5.2 hrs = .216 days
       k_d = ln2 ÷ .216 days = 3.2 day^{-1}
       k_s = $k_d P_{ss}$ = 3.2 day^{-1} x 5.94 x 10^2 pm/g = 1,900 pm/g/day

[b] Mouse

143

proteins are arrived at because of differences in the
relationship between rates of synthesis and degradation
during development and not because of the values for
$S(\infty)$ or $L(\infty)$. Thus, it can be seen in Figs. 1, 2 and
3 that during the developmental period between 12 and
40 days after birth, while rates of synthesis and
degradation are approaching steady state values, the
pyruvate kinase levels increase by 140, 450, and 2300
picomoles per gram in heart, liver and skeletal muscle,
respectively. This analysis shows why the adult level
of pyruvate kinase is 5 to 6 fold greater in rat skeletal muscle than in liver or heart while the rates of
synthesis of the enzyme in the adult animal are virtually the same in the three tissues (Table I). When
P has reached steady state, equation 4 shows that the
rate constant for degradation, $L(\infty)$, may be obtained
by dividing the rate constant for synthesis, $S(\infty)$, by
the steady state protein level $P(\infty)$. The rate constant for degradation is thus an indication of the
relative turnover and since half-life is derived
directly from this constant it becomes clear why rat
skeletal muscle pyruvate kinase has a half-life of
21.6 days while rat liver pyruvate kinase has a half-
life of 3.5 days (Table I). Steady state levels of
enzymes are not necessarily related to their turnover;
as an example, consider tyrosine amino transferase and
glyceraldehyde phosphate dehydrogenase (Table II).
Although the steady state amounts of these two enzymes
in rat liver are roughly the same, their absolute
steady state turnover and their value of k_d differ by
almost 50 fold (Table II). Further consideration of
Table II indicates that comparison of half-lives alone
as a measure of turnover gives a picture entirely different from that derived from a comparison of the
absolute rate of turnover. When the molecules are
compared on a molar basis, it is seen that even though
rat liver serine dehydratase has a half-life of 5.2
hours, its absolute turnover is about 3-fold less
than rat liver aldolase with a half-life of 67 hours.

Short half-lives have often been associated with
high rates of turnover, and many authors have assumed

that this is a consistent relationship, and that regulation of steady state levels is achieved strictly by regulation of half-life. That this is not necessarily so is shown by the following examples. Rat liver tyrosine amino transferase and serine dehydratase levels change quickly and markedly as a consequence of alterations in diet and certain hormone levels. It might be inferred from this that such changes were related to the fast relative and absolute turnover of these enzymes (Table II). However, it is also well known that rat liver pyruvate kinase levels change just as quickly and markedly as a result of dietary and hormonal changes, and yet the relative and absolute turnover of this enzyme could hardly be considered fast compared to tyrosine amino transferase or serine dehydratase. In addition, there is no evidence to indicate that rat liver aldolase levels fluctuate in response to dietary or hormonal changes in spite of its extremely fast absolute turnover.

In summary, we have presented a method for studying protein turnover during times when intracellular protein levels are changing and have demonstrated the applicability of the method to the specific situation of changing pyruvate kinase levels in rat heart, liver, and skeletal muscle during postnatal development. Analysis of protein turnover in situations other than steady state is instructive because, as these studies indicate, such analyses reveal that even though steady state levels of different proteins may differ by large amounts, their rates of synthesis or degradation may be the same. Conversely, these studies also show how steady state levels of different proteins may be the same when their rates of synthesis or degradation differ greatly.

Acknowledgements

Aided by Grant BC-50A from the American Cancer Society and by Grant CA-12808 from the United States Public Health Service.

References

1. Schimke, R. T. & Doyle, D.   Ann. Rev. Biochem. 39: 929 (1970).
2. Ciba Foundation Symposium 9 (new series), "Protein Turnover", Wolstenholme, G. and O'Connor, M., eds. Eslevier, Amsterdam, (1973).
3. Greengard, O.   Essays in Biochem. 7: 159 (1971).
4. Murison, G.   Develop. Biol. 20: 518 (1969).
5. Haining, J. L., Legan, J. S., Lovell, W. J. J. Geront. 25: 205 (1970).
6. Ove, P., Obenrader, M. & Lansing, A.   Biochem. Biophys. Acta 277: 211 (1972).
7. Phillipidis, H., Hanson, R. W., Reshef, L., Hopgood, M. F. & Ballard, F. J.   Biochem. J. 126: 1127 (1972).
8. Zilversmit, D. B., Entenmam, C. & Fishler, M. C. J. Gen. Physiol. 26: 325 (1943).
9. Zilversmit, D. B.   Nature 175: 863 (1955).
10. Reiner, J. M.   Arch. Biochem. Biophys. 46: 53 (1953).
11. Osterman, J., Fritz, P. J. & Wuntch, T.   J. Biol. Chem. 248: 1011 (1973).
12. Kenney, F. T.   J. Biol. Chem. 237: 3495 (1962).
13. Kenney, F. T.   Science 156: 525 (1967).
14. Nakagawa, H., Kimura, H. & Miura, S.   Biochem. Biophys. Res. Commun. 28: 359 (1967).
15. Nakagawa, H., & Kimura, H.   J. Biochem. 66: 669 (1969).
16. Jost, J. P., Khairallah, E. A. & Pitot, H. C. J. Biol. Chem. 243: 3057 (1968).
17. Nakanishi, S. & Numa, S.   Europ. J. Biochem. 16: 161 (1970).
18. Kuehl, L. & Sumsion, E. N.   J. Biol. Chem. 245: 6616 (1970).
19. Doyle, D. & Schimke, R. T.   J. Biol. Chem. 244: 5449 (1969).
20. Doyle, D.   J. Biol. Chem. 246: 4965 (1971).
21. Fritz, P. J., White, E. L., Pruitt, K. M. & Vesell, E. S.   Biochemistry 12: 4034 (1973).

STUDIES ON DEGRADATION OF TYROSINE AMINOTRANSFERASE IN LIVER AND HEPATOMA CELLS

Francis T. Kenney, Ronald W. Johnson, and Kai-Lin Lee

Carcinogenesis Program, Biology Division
Oak Ridge National Laboratory
Oak Ridge, Tennessee 37830

Introduction

The tyrosine aminotransferase of rat liver was among the earliest known hormonally-inducible enzymes (1) and was the first for which it was demonstrated that increased activity following hormone treatment is the result of increased synthesis of the enzyme (2). In the course of this earlier work it was quickly recognized that the enzyme undergoes rapid turnover in vivo, both from the kinetics of enzyme change during induction and from direct immunochemical-isotopic measurements. These early measurements indicated a half-life of 3 to 4 hours, but as techniques improved it became apparent that the true half-life in rat liver is about 1.5 to 2 hours (Fig. 1). Fortunately for those who chose to use this enzyme as a model for the study of regulation in mammalian cells, the tyrosine aminotransferase and its hormonal regulation is virtually identical in cultured rat hepatoma cells and in liver, and its rate of degradation is also remarkably constant in liver cells and in their malignant counterparts cultured in vitro. We have carried out a variety of studies aimed at gaining understanding of the molecular basis for the unusually rapid turnover of this enzyme, and shall summarize some of them here.

147

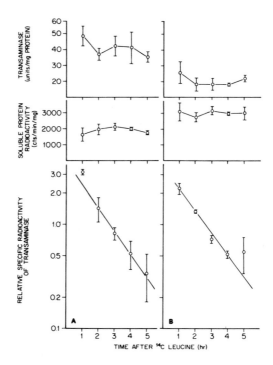

Figure 1: Turnover of rat liver tyrosine aminotransferase <u>in vivo</u>. Data are mean ± SD for 3
animals at each point. Male rats were adrenal-
ectomized and fasted for 24 hr, then given (at
zero time) 50 μl of (^{14}C)leucine intraperitoneally. The lower plots are the ratio of radioactivity in the enzyme (determined by immune precipitation after partial purification) to that in
the soluble proteins. From Kenney (3).

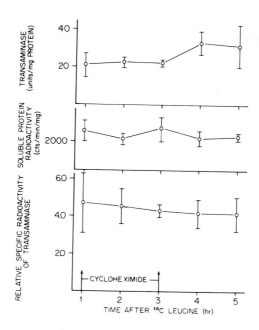

Figure 2: Inhibition of turnover in cycloheximide-
treated rats. Details as in Fig. 1 except that
animals killed after the first hr received cycloheximide (100 μg/100 g) intraperitoneally at 1 hr
and again at 3 hr after (^{14}C)-leucine. From
Kenney (3).

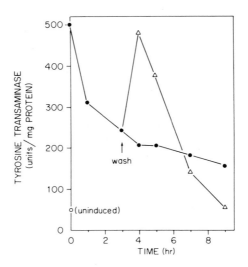

Figure 3: Effect of cycloheximide on turnover of
tyrosine aminotransferase in cultured H35 cells.
Cells were pre-induced with hydrocortisone to
the induced steady state, then cycloheximide
(5 µg/ml) was added. Solid circles: no further
manipulations. Triangles: at the point indicated
cycloheximide was removed by washing the cells.

Results and Discussion

<u>Apparent requirement for protein synthesis.</u> The results of early studies on the effect of inhibitors of protein synthesis on hormonal induction of tyrosine aminotransferase, while showing clearly that induction was blocked by these inhibitors, were puzzling in another aspect: if turnover is rapid, why does the basal level of enzyme not fall when enzyme synthesis is blocked? Among the possible explanations are: (1) turnover rates of "induced" and "basal" enzymes are different; (2) synthesis of the basal level of enzyme is not affected by antibiotic inhibitors of protein synthesis; or (3) degradation as well as synthesis is blocked by these inhibitors. We approached this question directly in experiments in which rats were given isotopic amino acids in a fashion known to label liver proteins (including tyrosine aminotransferase) for a period of 30 to 45 min; measurements of radioactivity in proteins beginning at 60 min thus constitute a classical "chase" analysis of degradation rate. If cycloheximide (or puromycin), in amounts sufficient to block protein synthesis more or less completely, was given during the chase, radioactivity in tyrosine aminotransferase remained essentially constant (Fig. 2). This clear indication that aminotransferase degradation is blocked when protein synthesis stops was later confirmed in cultured hepatoma cells (Fig. 3), where the greater precision attainable made it apparent that degradation proceeds at the normal rate for a period of about 1 hour, then slows and stops about 2 hours after cessation of protein synthesis.

Comparable effects on aminotransferase degradation are observed when very high concentrations of actinomycin are added to this medium of cultured hepatoma cells, whether synthesis of the enzyme is induced or not (4-6). In cells in which enzyme synthesis has been elevated by prior treatment with hydrocortisone, this effect of actinomycin leads to an interesting phenomenon; the enzyme level increases, sometimes markedly, instead of declining as expected (7). This effect, unfortunately given the misnomer "superinduction".

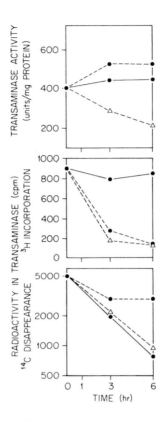

Figure 4: Effects of high and low concentrations
of actinomycin on aminotransferase synthesis and
degradation in H35 cells. Cells were preinduced
with hydrocortisone to the induced steady state
before experiments began. At zero time actinomycin
was added at 0.2 μg/ml (triangles), 5 μg/ml (solid
circles, broken line), or none (solid circles,
solid line). Top panel, enzyme levels; middle
panel, pulse-labeling measurements of rate of
enzyme synthesis; lower panel, chase measurements
of rate of enzyme degradation. From Lee et al.
(6).

is not due to further increase in synthesis but, instead, to inhibition of degradation (4,6,8). As shown in Fig. 4, synthesis of tyrosine aminotransferase is actually inhibited by both low and high concentrations of actinomycin, but the enzyme level is increased only by the high concentration which blocks degradation of the enzyme. The increase in enzyme level observed under these conditions can be understood in the requirement for prior induction by hydrocortisone. Kinetic and inhibitor studies show, albeit indirectly, that the steroid promotes synthesis of aminotransferase mRNA, which has a half-life of about 2 hours (4-6). When further synthesis of this mRNA is blocked by actinomycin enzyme synthesis begins to decline. However, because of the finite lifetime of the mRNA, synthesis is still at a high rate for the first few hours after actinomycin treatment; during this interval degradation slows and stops, and hence the enzyme level rises. The high levels of actinomycin required to block aminotransferase degradation have marked inhibitory effects on protein synthesis in these cells, so we suspect that this effect of actinomycin is simply another indication of an apparent requirement for protein synthesis in degradation of this enzyme.

We have used the term "apparent" in describing this requirement because it is not yet understood. One interpretation could be that some cellular component whose level is dependent on functioning of the translational apparatus, is required for aminotransferase degradation. We suggested (3) that this may be a degradative enzyme, highly specific (since degradation of other inducible enzymes is not blocked by these inhibitors) and itself undergoing rapid turnover (since degradation ceases about two hours after protein synthesis stops). However, a direct search for such an enzyme has been fruitless, as have all of many attempts to develop a cell-free system in which aminotransferase degradation can be observed. Further, this mechanism now seems rather illogical; if rapid degradation of tyrosine aminotransferase requires a protein which is itself degraded even more rapidly, then what controls degradation of that protein? One is led to imagine an

153

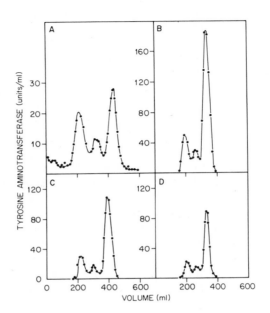

Figure 5: Multiple forms of rat liver tyrosine
aminotransferase after hormonal induction. The
animals were killed at 2 p.m., 3 hr after intraperitoneal administration of hormones. (A) untreated;
(B) hydrocortisone, 1 mg/100 g; (C) dibutyryl cyclic
AMP, 6 mg/100 g; (D) insulin, 2.5 units/100 g plus
glucose. From Johnson et al. (13).

endless series of proteins, each turning over more
rapidly than the preceding one, and all devoted to
controlling the rate of turnover of tyrosine aminotransferase. Rather than disappearance from the cell
of something required for aminotransferase degradation, perhaps something accumulates in cells not making proteins (e.g., charged tRNAs) which inhibits the
degradative process. As yet there are no definitive
data to enable choosing between these alternatives.

Multiple Enzyme Forms

In recent years several reports have appeared of
multiple forms of tyrosine aminotransferase, distinguishable by electrophoresis or ion exchange chromatography and thus differing in net charge (9-12). We
found that the three forms separated by CM-Sephadex
chromatography were otherwise indistinguishable by
several criteria, including coenzyme content, heat
denaturation rates, approximate molecular weight, and
immunological reactivity (13). These findings, especially the immunological identity of the three forms,
indicates that they are not the products of different
genes. Further, the specific activities of each of
the three forms, when the enzyme was highly purified,
were found to be essentially identical. What, then,
is the biological significance in having three forms
of the same enzyme, differing (apparently) only in
net charge?

Other investigators approaching this question concluded that the different hormonal inducers of tyrosine aminotransferase (glucocorticoids, insulin, cyclic
AMP) enhance the cellular levels of specific forms of
the enzyme (9-11). Since this conclusion was at vari-
ance with the results of analyses of hormonal induction in our laboratory (5,6) we reinvestigated the
question, confining our measurements to that portion
of each induction cycle when the enzyme level is increasing. Our results (Fig. 5) show that, when the
analysis is made at a time when induced enzyme synthesis is proceeding at maximal rate, each of the hormonal inducers promotes specifically that form which
is eluted last from CM-Sephadex, and which we called

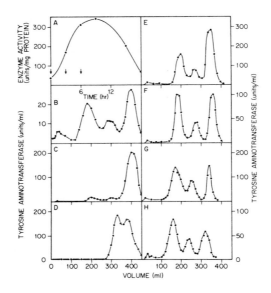

Figure 6: Changes in the patterns of multiple forms
after hydrocortisone treatment. (A) aminotransferase activity as a function of time, hydrocortisone given at times indicated by arrows. Pattern
of multiple forms at B, zero time; (C) 3 hr; (D)
6 hr; (E) 9 hr; (F) 12 hr; (G) 15 hr; (H) 18 hr.
From Johnson et al. (13).

Form I. From this and other results (13) we concluded that Form I is the immediate product of translation, the others arising from it by post-translational modifications which confer greater negative charge on the protein.

It is particularly interesting to note the changes in pattern of the multiple forms during the time course of induction and deinduction (Fig. 6). Under the conditions of hydrocortisone treatment we employed, the enzyme level rises sharply for a period of about 6 hours, then levels off as the inducing stimulus disappears due to metabolism of hydrocortisone. After about 9 hours induced synthesis ceases, degradation becomes predominant and the enzyme level begins a rapid decay to return to the basal level at about 18 hours (Fig. 6A). In the earliest phase of this cycle, when inducted synthesis is maximal, virtually no conversion of Form I to Forms II and III is observed (Fig. 6C). It is especially significant that Levitan & Webb have shown that degradation of the enzyme is essentially completely blocked during this phase of the induction cycle (14). After 6 hours, when degradation is resumed as the system approaches a new steady state, Form II becomes predominant (Fig. 6D). At 9, 12, 15 and 18 hours after hormone, when degradation is dominant, a progressively larger fraction of the enzyme appears as Forms II and III (Fig. 6E to H). To summarize, when induced synthesis is dominant and, according to Levitan & Webb, degradation is inhibited, the enzyme is largely present as Form I; when degradation is paramount, most of the enzyme has undergone posttranslational modification to Forms II and III.

These data suggest to us that the significance of the multiple forms of tyrosine aminotransferase (otherwise without apparent significance) relates to the rapid turnover of this enzyme, i.e., that posttranslational modification may be preliminary to degradation of the enzyme.

If this tentative conclusion is correct, the nature of the modifications of the enzyme assumes increased importance, for therein may be the key to the cellular

157

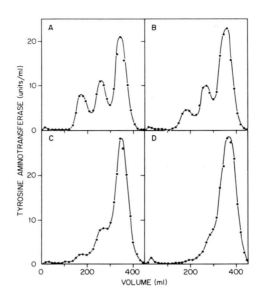

Figure 7: Conversion of the multiple forms to Form I
<u>in</u> <u>vitro</u>. Aliquots of the supernatant fraction of
liver from a hydrocortisone-treated rat were
chromatographed without incubation (A) or after
incubation at 25° for 5 min (B), 15 min (C), or
30 min (D). Total aminotransferase units were
4170 (A), 4306 (B), 4260 (C) and 4180 (D). From
Johnson et al. (13).

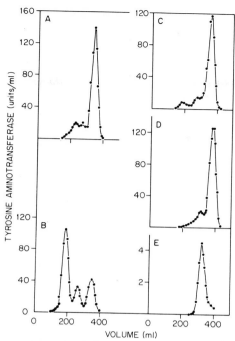

Figure 8: Interconversion of the multiple forms in the presence of potassium cyanate in vitro. Aliquots of supernatant fractions were chromatographed after incubation at 25° as follows: (A), crude homogenate, not incubated; (B), crude homogenate, 10 mM potassium cyanate; (C), soluble fraction, 10 mM potassium cyanate; (D), crude homogenate, incubated with no addition; (D) purified Form I, 5 mM potassium cyanate. From Johnson et al. (13).

TABLE I   INCORPORATION OF ^{32}P INTO THE MULTIPLE FORMS
OF TYROSINE AMINOTRANSFERASE

Enzyme Form	Radioactivity(A)	Enzyme Activity(B)	A/B x 100
	cpm	units	
I	1,050	24,615	4.3
II	1,500	8,594	17.5
III	500	1,400	35.7

H35 cells were treated with hydrocortisone for 24 hr prior to addition of 40 µCi/ml of ^{32}Pi. Two hr later cells were collected and the soluble fraction was chromatographed to separate the multiple forms. After concentration each form was precipitated with anti aminotransferase antiserum.

159

mechanisms controlling degradation. We have developed several leads to this question, some of the conflicting, and do not yet have a definitive answer. It is clear that the modifications converting Form I to Forms II and III can be readily reversed simply by incubation of soluble fractions of liver at 25° (Fig. 7). This reaction appears to require a soluble component (enzyme?) that does not bind to CM-Sephadex, since it does not occur with enzyme preparations subjected to this chromatographic procedure. The ease with which this shift occurs in vitro obviously means that to obtain valid patterns of the in vivo distribution requires very careful and rapid analyses, and that this may account for much of the confusion in the literature concerning the multiple forms of tyrosine aminotransferase. The nature of the demodification reaction exemplified in Fig. 7 is now being investigated.

A variety of biochemical additions and incubation conditions were explored in an attempt to develop an in vitro system in which conversion of Form I to Forms II and III could be observed. Reproducible conversion could be demonstrated in vitro when liver homogenates were incubated with potassium cyanate under conditions in which carbamylation of enzyme amino groups could occur (Fig. 8). Such a reaction would reduce net positive charge and could account for the chromatographic shifts observed. This conversion appeared to require a particulate component, since it did not occur in soluble fractions or with purified enzyme, but its mechanism and especially its significance have not yet been further clarified.

A second possible mechanism by which posttranslational modification could produce enzyme forms carrying increased net negative charge lies in the recent finding that tyrosine aminotransferase is a phosphoprotein (15). Removal of much of the enzyme-bound phosphate did not change enzyme activity appreciably, which is consistent with the fact that modification does not appear to change catalytic capacity of the enzyme. Further, preliminary analyses of the phosphate content of the three forms (Table I) indicate that Form II contains 4 times as much phosphate as Form I, and III is labeled twice as heavily as II.

At the moment, then, we are left with two equally plausible and probably mutually exclusive mechanisms to account for the posttranslational modification of tyrosine aminotransferase, and without any indication of a potential role of these reactions in degradation of the enzyme. And, to complicate matters further, it is not possible to relate, even conceptually, either of these mechanisms with the apparent requirement for protein synthesis in aminotransferase degradation.

General Discussion

Most papers written in the last decade on the question of protein turnover in mammalian cells begin with what has become almost a ritual exposition of (a) the importance of the problem, and (b) the deplorable state of ignorance of the cellular mechanisms involved. We disagree with neither of these attitudes, especially as is perhaps apparent from the preceding paragraph, the second one. Our approach, which has been to analyze turnover of a single enzyme which is degraded rapidly and is otherwise a convenient model, would appear to have developed more questions than it has answers.

Perhaps part of the problem is that we have not yet developed reagents capable of detecting specific proteins in the course of their degradation. Our methods for detecting tyrosine aminotransferase have been limited to two; assay of its catalytic activity and of its reaction with specific antibody. We have assumed that these are measuring different parameters, but have always been struck by the precision with which the activity level of a given liver or hepatoma preparation is matched by its antigen content. Thus under none of the physiological conditions we have employed in the study of this enzyme have we been able to detect, for example, a form of the enzyme which has lost activity but retains immunological reactivity. Recent experiments suggest that the reason for this is that the two methods may actually be measuring the same thing, i.e., a given conformation which is required for enzyme activity and is also the basis for antigenicity. If confirmed, this would explain our previous inability to detect partially degraded enzyme, and would suggest that antisera against a variety of denatured or degraded preparations might be more useful in. the study of intracellular turnover of specific proteins.

References

1. Lin, E. C. C. & Knox, W. E. Biochim. Biophys. Acta 26, 85 (1957).
2. Kenney, F. T. J. Biol. Chem. 237, 3495 (1962).
3. Kenney, F. T. Science 156, 525 (1967).
4. Reel, J. R. & Kenney, F. T. Proc. Nat. Acad. Sci. U.S.A. 61, 200 (1968).
5. Reel, J. R., Lee, K.-L. & Kenney, F. T. J. Biol. Chem. 245, 5800 (1970).
6. Lee, K. -L., Reel, J. R. & Kenney, F. T. J. Biol. Chem. 245, 5806 (1970).
7. Tomkins, G. M., Thompson, E. G., Hayashi, S., Gelehrter, I., Granner, D. & Peterkofsky, B. Cold Spring Harbor Symp. Quant. Biol. 31, 349 (1966).
8. Kenney, F. T., Lee, K.-L., Stiles, C. D. & Fritz, J. E. Nature New Biol. 246, 208 (1973).
9. Holt, P. G. & Oliver, I. T. Fed. Eur. Biochem. Soc. Lett. 5, 89 (1969).
10. Holt, P. G. & Oliver, I. T. Fed. Eur. Biochem. Soc. Lett. 8, 99 (1970).
11. Iwasaki, Y. & Pitot, H. C. Life Sci. 10, 1071 (1971).
12. Blake, R. L. & Bonner, J. Biochem. Biophys. Res. Commun. 41, 1443 (1970).
13. Johnson, R. W., Roberson, L. E. & Kenney, F. T. J. Biol. Chem. 248, 4521 (1973).
14. Levitan, I. B. & Webb, T. E. J. Mol. Biol. 48, 339 (1970).
15. Lee, K.-L. & Nickol, J. M. J. Biol. Chem. in press.

INTRACELLULAR TURNOVER OF AN ALTERED ENZYME

Ronald W. Johnson and Francis T. Kenney

Department of Pharmacology
New York University School of Medicine
New York, New York 10016

and

Carcinogenesis Program
Biology Division
Oak Ridge National Laboratory
Oak Ridge, Tennessee 37830

Introduction

There is an extensive literature relating susceptibility of proteins to proteolytic attack and the extent
of their denaturation (for a review see Schimke [1]),
and it is widely assumed that these observations are
relevant to intracellular turnover of proteins. Indeed, as shown by Goldberg, E. coli proteins which
contain analogs of amino acids are degraded more
rapidly than normal proteins in vivo (2) as well as by
various proteases in vitro (3). We wished to analyze
further the concept that labile conformers of a protein molecule are selectively degraded in vivo, particularly by examining the relationship between stability of an identifiable protein (with enzymatic
activity) and its rate of intracellular turnover. To
do so, we devised conditions for synthesis in cultured
hepatoma cells of tyrosine aminotransferase containing
fluorinated derivatives of tryptophan, and asked whether
the turnover of the altered enzyme was changed. Details

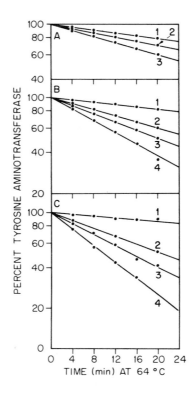

Figure 1: Thermal inactivation of tyrosine aminotransferase from cells treated with fluorotryptophan isomers. (A), DL-4-fluorotryptophan. Curve
1, native enzyme; 2, 0.1 mM; 3, 0.25 mM. (B), DL-
5-fluorotryptophan. Curve 1, native enzyme; 2,
0.1 mM; 3, 0.4 mM; 4, 1.0 mM. (C), DL-6-fluoro-
tryptophan. Curve 1, native enzyme; 2, 0.025 mM;
3, 0.10 mM; 4, 0.25 mM. From Johnson & Kenney (4).

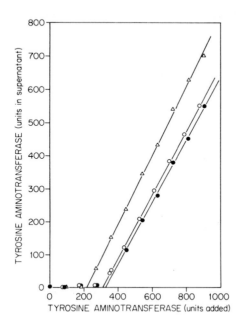

Figure 2: Immunochemical titration of aminotransferase from analog-treated cells and control cells. Solid circles, native enzyme; open circles, enzyme from cells treated with trifluoroleucine; triangles, enzyme from 5-fluorotryptophan-treated cells. From Johnson & Kenney (4).

of these experiments can be found in our original publication (4).

Results

Aminotransferase synthesis was induced (by hydrocortisone) in H35 cells incubated with a variety of amino acid analogs, and their capacity to alter the physical properties of the enzyme was monitored by heat stability measurements. Of the analogs tested, the fluorinated derivatives of tryptophan had the greatest effect on this parameter, and the degree of change in denaturation rate was dependent on concentration of the analog in the medium (Fig. 1). Incorporation of either 5-fluoro- or 6-fluorotryptophan into the enzyme resulted in markedly increased lability of the enzyme, and these derivatives were employed in subsequent experiments.

To determine if catalytic capacity of the enzyme was changed by analog incorporation, analog-treated and native enzymes were titrated with antiaminotransferase serum (Fig. 2). Varying amounts of the enzymes were reacted with sufficient antiserum to precipitate 330 units of the native enzyme. Enzyme from cells treated with trifluoroleucine, which did not alter sensitivity to heat, was similarly unchanged by this criterion. However, equivalence was reached with only 220 units of enzyme from fluorotryptophan-treated cells, indicating that the fluorotryptophan enzyme has, on the average, about two-thirds of the catalytic activity per molecule of the native enzyme.

Thus, by two criteria - heat stability and catalytic activity - it is apparent that fluorotryptophan is incorporated into the enzyme and significantly changes the physical properties of the enzyme. How does this change in structure affect intracellular turnover of the enzyme?

To answer this question we devised a double-isotope experiment that enabled measurement of turnover rates of both native and analog-containing enzyme in the same cells, thereby excluding the possibility that analog treatment alters some cellular component other

166

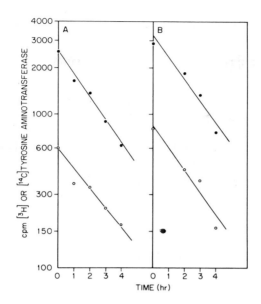

Figure 3: Effect of incorporation of 6-fluorotrypto-
phan on aminotransferase turnover _in vivo_. (A),
turnover of analog-treated and native enzymes from
cells treated with 6-fluorotryptophan. Solid
circles, ^{3}H-labeled, analog-containing enzyme;
open circles, ^{14}C-labeled native enzyme. (B),
turnover of native enzyme in control cells.
Solid circles, ^{3}H-labeled; open circles, [14]C-
labeled native enzyme.

than the aminotransferase. Briefly, enzyme synthesis was elevated to a high rate by treatment with hydrocortisone, then native enzyme was labeled with ^{14}C by exposure of the cultures to [^{14}C]valine for 2 hr. The medium was then replaced with one containing [^{3}H] valine and 0.1 mM 6-fluorotryptophan; during this 2 hr interval analog-containing enzyme also containing ^{3}H was formed. Flasks were harvested when the medium was changed to one containing no isotope (zero time) and at each subsequent hour for 4 hr, and the content of each isotope in the enzyme was determined as previously described (5). A control experiment utilizing both isotopes but without fluorotryptophan was run in similar fashion. The results of the chase measurements of enzyme turnover in these cells (Fig. 3) show clearly that the analog-containing enzyme (^{3}H-labeled), Fig. 3A) is degraded at the same rate as the native enzyme. Heat stability measurements confirmed that the cells analyzed in Fig. 3A contained two populations of aminotransferase, one being 5 times more sensitive to heat than the native enzyme. Thus an analog-induced change in the physical properties of tyrosine aminotransferase, sufficient to cause marked change in heat stability and catalytic activity, did not result in a change in the rate of degradation of the enzyme in vivo.

Discussion

In the course of these experiments, we examined fluorotryptophan-containing enzymes for sensitivity to proteases (e.g., trypsin) and found it to be only marginally more sensitive than the native enzyme. However, we have tended to discount the significance of this result, since the native enzyme is remarkably stable to proteolytic attack in vitro, i.e., there is no correlation of this parameter with the remarkable lability of tyrosine aminotransferase in vivo. By the criteria we have employed, it is clear that a marked change in physical properties of the enzyme did not change its intracellular rate of turnover.

This result raises several issues, among them the validity of the view that physical properties of a protein are rate-limiting in its intracellular turnover. The apparent disparity between this result and those reported by Goldberg (2,3) may reflect the fact that we have analyzed turnover of a complete and, although altered appreciably, intact protein which retains both antigenic and enzyme activity. Experiments in which turnover of total cell proteins is analyzed may be biased by the presence of proteins which are incomplete or totally altered by analog incorporation, and these may well be selectively degraded in the cell.

A second important question arising from this and other studies on turnover rates of specific proteins is this: to what extent are we justified in equating "turnover" with "degradation"? As described in another chapter, our measurements of intracellular turnover rate measure disappearance of an entity detectable in terms of its enzyme activity and immunological reactivity; it is not, in fact, known that the protein is _degraded_ at this rate. Thus, the failure of analog-induced change in physical structure to alter intracellular turnover rate may be another indication that this is not actually the rate at which the enzyme is degraded, but rather that this rate reflects some reaction which renders the enzyme undetectable by the usual methods. The physiological significance of intracellular turnover rates of specific proteins is unquestionable; the enzyme, as a functional entity, is removed from the cell at that rate. However, the nature of the chemical reactions which determine these rates remains elusive.

References

1. Schimke, R. T. in Mammalian Protein Metabolism, (H. N. Munro, ed.), Vol. 4, p. 177, Academic Press, New York (1970).
2. Goldberg, A. L. Proc. Nat. Acad. Sci. U.S.A. 69, 422 (1972).

3. Goldberg, A. L.   Proc. Nat. Acad. Sci. U.S.A. 69, 2640.

4. Johnson, R. W. & Kenney, F. T.   J. Biol. Chem. 248, 4528 (1973).

5. Lee, K.-L. & Kenney, F. T.   Acta Endocrinol. 153, (Suppl) 109 (1970).

Mechanisms for Regulation of
Protein Turnover

ON THE PROPERTIES AND MECHANISMS OF PROTEIN TURNOVER

Robert T. Schimke

Department of Biological Sciences
Stanford University
Stanford, California 94305

Knowledge of the events of regulation of protein synthesis has increased rapidly in the past two decades, in large part as a result of the ready availability of mutants in prokaryotes. In contrast, understanding of the processes for breakdown of cell proteins has lagged, despite the fact that this process is equally important in the total economy of an organism or population of organisms (or cells). Although the existence of continual protein turnover was promulgated by the classical work of Rudolf Schoenheimer and his colleagues in "The Dynamic State of Body Constituents" (1) published in 1942, awareness of the importance of protein degradation has developed increasingly in the past 10 years as a result of the appreciation that control of degradation can be important in determining the levels of a number of specific proteins (see Schimke & Doyle [2] for examples) in animal tissues. In addition, there is an increasing awareness of the existence of protein turnover in prokaryotes. Thus, prior to the last decade, it was generally accepted that protein turnover was insignificant in growing bacteria, most notably Escherichia coli (3,4). More recently, various investigators have shown that protein degradation occurs in both growing and non-growing bacteria, but that the rates and proportions of protein subject to degradation differ in the two growth states (5,6). In fact, it appears that the general properties of turnover are quite similar

in prokaryotes and eukaryotes, and hence both types of
systems can provide information about this important
biological process. Thus, acknowledgement of the generality of protein turnover, as well as the increasing
understanding of its role in biological regulation,
has led to a marked interest in understanding this
important biological process.

This article is basically a status report on certain aspects of protein turnover. Firstly, I shall
deal with the general properties of protein turnover
and use specific examples from the currently most
studied system, the intact rat liver. Secondly, I
shall raise questions concerning the mechanism and
regulation of protein degradation.

General Properties of Degradation of Protein

1. Turnover is extensive. Studies of Swick (7),
Buchanan (8), and Schimke (9) have shown that essentially all proteins of rat liver undergo continual
replacement. Buchanan (8) estimated that about 70%
of rat liver protein was replaced every 4-5 days from
the dietary source.

2. Turnover is largely intracellular. Turnover
includes synthesis and secretion of proteins, cell
replacement, as well as intracellular synthesis and
degradation. The life span of hepatic cells is of
the order of 160-400 days (10,11). Hence, the extensive turnover occurring in 4-5 days indicates that
protein turnover in liver is largely intracellular.

3. There is a marked heterogeneity of rate of
replacement of different proteins (enzymes). Table
I gives a representative listing of rates of degradation of various enzymes of rat liver. The variation
of half-lives is remarkable, ranging from 10 minutes
for ornithine decarboxylase to 16 days for LDH_5 and
NAD glycohydrolase. There is no correlation between
half-lives and the cell fraction from which the enzyme
is isolated. For instance, δ-aminolevulinate synthetase and ornithine aminotransferase, both of which
are associated with mitochondria, have half-lives of
60 min and 1 day respectively, whereas total mitochondrial protein has a half-life of 4-5 days. Equally

174

remarkable are the marked differences in half-lives of
enzymes associated with the internal membranes of rat
liver, ranging from 2 hrs for HMG-CoA reductase to 16
days for NAD glycohydrolase.

In addition, the rates at which specific proteins
are degraded varies with the physiological state.
Schimke et al. (17) showed that administration of
tryptophan to animals results in accumulation of tryptophan oxygenase, an effect that results from continued
enzyme synthesis with cessation of the normally occuring rapid degradation (half-life of 2 hrs.). Schimke
(9) also demonstrated that arginase accumulates in rat
liver during starvation as a result of decreased degradation in the presence of continued synthesis. Majerus
& Kilburn (24) as well as Numa (these proceedings)
have shown that starvation increases the rate of degradation of acetyl CoA carboxylase.

The conclusion to be made from such studies is that
there is a continual process in which the total complement of any given enzyme is replaced at different rates,
and those rates can be altered by a variety of physiological conditions.

4. The degradation of an enzyme molecule, once
synthesized, is a random process. This conclusion
is based on the essentially universal finding that
the decay of isotopically labeled enzyme following a
single isotope administration follows first-order
kinetics (2). The most likely interpretation of this
finding is that once a newly synthesized enzyme molecule enters a pool of like molecules, its chance of
being degraded (or otherwise removed from the pool of
like molecules) is a random process. Thus, there is
no evidence for an accumulation of damage, i.e., aging,
to explain why a given enzyme molecule is degraded.

5. There is a correlation between the size of
proteins and their rates of degradation. Dehlinger
& Schimke (27) first showed that large proteins have
greater relative rates of degradation than small proteins, as measured by the double-isotope method of
Arias et al. (25). Figure 1 shows this correlation
for rat liver "soluble" proteins. This same correlation holds for proteins of organelles, including

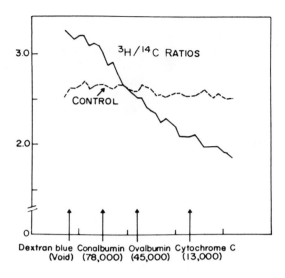

Figure 1. Fractionation of rat liver supernatant proteins on Sephadex G-200 in the presence of 0.1% sodium dodecyl sulfate. Male white Sprague-Dawley rats weighing 100-120 g each were given 100 µCi of ^{14}C-leucine in 2 ml of 0.85% NaCl ip. Four days later the animal was given 250 µCi of ^{3}H-leucine and sacrificed by decapitation 4 hours later. In a control experiment, an animal was given 50 µCi of ^{14}C-leucine and 250 µCi of ^{3}H-leucine simultaneously and sacrificed 4 hours later. The homogenate was centrifuged at $105,000g_{max}$ for 1 hour and the supernatant fraction (4 ml) was passed through a Sephadex G-25 column, 1.5 x 20 cm, equilibrated with the above buffer, to remove free amino acids. The column eluate to which SDS was added to a final concentration of 0.1% was sonicated for 30 seconds and a sample containing about 30 mg of protein was then applied to a Sephadex G-200 column. By this method, high $^3H/^{14}C$ ratios indicate rapid turnover.

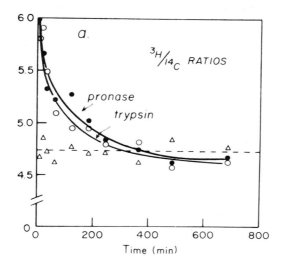

<u>Figure 2</u>. Degradation of rat liver soluble proteins <u>in vitro</u>. Double-labeled soluble proteins were prepared from rat liver as described in Fig. 1. The final soluble protein concentration was about 15 mg/ml. Pronase or trypsin was added as a 1 mg/ml solution in distilled water to a final concentration of 100 μg/ml. The digestion was allowed to proceed at 20°C and 100-μl aliquots were removed at various times and mixed with 100 μl of 20% TCA in 400-μl plastic microfuge tubes (Beckman) The tubes were centrifuged for 2 minutes in a Beckman model 152 micro-fuge ($15,000g_{max}$). The upper 100 μl of each soluble fraction were dissolved in 0.5 ml of NCS solublizer and counted in a toluene-based scintillation fluid. $^3H/^{14}C$ ratios of acid soluble fractions were determined when double-labeled soluble proteins were incubated with either pronase (●--●) or trypsin (0--0). The dotted line (Δ--Δ) indicates the results of a control experiment using soluble proteins which had received both ^3H- and ^{14}C-leucine 4 hours prior to sacrifice.

proteins associated with chromatin (28) and membranes (29), as well as cytoplasmic proteins from a variety of tissues (30). In addition, there is a correlation between the in vivo rate of degradation of cytoplasmic rat liver proteins and the capacity of trypsin and pronase to degrade proteins. As shown in Fig. 2, with proteins that have been doubly labeled in vivo to differentially label proteins with rapid turnover, i.e., high $^3H^{14}C$ ratios (25), digestion of the isolated proteins in vitro by pronase preferentially releases to a soluble form radioactivity with a high $^3H/^{14}C$ ratio, indicating that proteins that turn over rapidly in the intact animal are preferentially degraded in vitro. The preferential degradation of these proteins appears to be a function of their conformation state, since when the proteins are first unfolded by denaturation in urea and the sulfhydryl groups blocked by aminoethylation, the preferential degradation is not observed (30). In addition, these same workers showed that large cytoplasmic proteins are degraded more rapidly than small proteins by various proteases (Fig. 3).

Such studies have led us to propose that the correlation of size and rate of degradation is based on the overall greater chance of a larger protein being "hit" by a protease, producing an initial rate-limiting peptide bond cleavage, with subsequent unfolding and rapid degradation to amino acids. The unexpected finding that intracellular organelles are not turning over as units also leads us to propose that there is a continual association-dissociation of assembled macromolecular structures, and that degradation occurs in the dissociated state. This suggestion has been supported by studies of Tweto, Dehlinger & Larrabee (31) showing that the dissimilar subunits of the fatty acid synthetase complex of rat liver are turning over at different rates, with large subunits turning over more rapidly than small subunit components. This suggestion is also consistent with the finding that the protease-susceptible form of apo-ornithine transaminase is a disaggregated form (Katanuma et al., these proceedings).

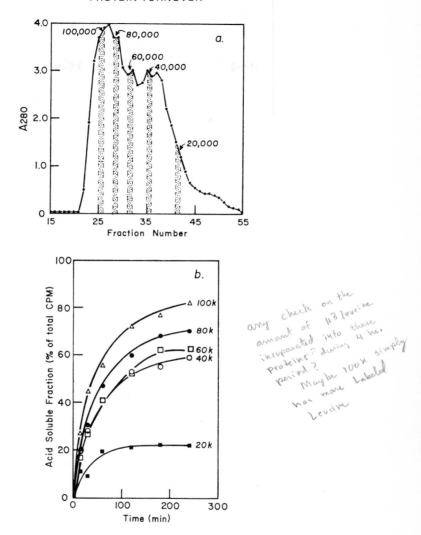

Figure 3. Fractionation of rat liver soluble proteins on Sephadex G-100 in the absence of SDS, and in vitro degradation of rat liver soluble proteins of specific molecular size ranges. A rat was given 1 mCi of [³H]leucine and then killed 4 hours later. Liver soluble proteins were prepared as described in the legend of Fig. 1. The soluble proteins were then fractionated on Sephadex G-100. Fractions containing proteins of specific molecular size (shaded areas of Fig. 3 A) were collected based on the eultion volumes of protein markers of known molecular weights (elution positions not shown), and were adjusted by dilution to the same protein concentration (2.0 mg per ml). Proteins of each molecular size range were digested with Pronase (100 µg/ml) at 20°. See reference 30 for details.

The correlation between size and degradation rate deals with proteins generally, and it is not surprising that it may not hold for selected proteins. For instance, arginase, tyrosine aminotransferase, all have similar molecular weights, but turn over at markedly different rates (see Table I). Such proteins likely have specific properties for stability, including cofactor association or different rates of dissociation into subunits that are important in the regulation of their degradation. Dice & Goldberg (32) have recently made correlations between rates of turnover of cytoplasmic proteins and their molecular size. Although they found little correlation between molecular size of the multimeric protein and turnover rate, they found a good correlation with subunit size, supporting the concept that proteins are more susceptible to degradation in a dissociated state. Again, it should be emphasized that insufficient numbers of specific enzymes have been studied to make a correlation for specific enzymes of the type that can be made for total cytoplasmic proteins.

On The Mechanisms of Protein Turnover in Animal Cells

As with any biochemical reaction, two components are necessary: (1) the substrate molecule, i.e., the protein to be degraded, and (2) the enzymatic apparatus involved in hydrolysis of peptide bonds. Either factor may be rate-limiting for protein degradation. Figure 4 depicts a number of possible regulatory processes that may be involved.

1. The properties of the protein molecule as a substrate for degradation. Protein molecules exist in a number of conformation states of varying degrees of detection. Thus, a protein molecule is subject to degradation only when it assumes certain conformations where susceptible peptide bonds are exposed. Heterogeneity of degradation rates would depend on the number and nature of particularly labile peptide bonds exposed in certain conformations. Obviously, the conformation state of a protein, including the state of aggregation, will depend on its interactions with a variety of ligands, including lipids (membrane proteins), cofactors,

TABLE I.

Half-lives of Specific Enzymes and Subcellular Fractions of Rat Liver

Enzymes	Half-life	Reference
Ornithine decarboxylase (soluble)	11 min	(12)
δ-Aminolevulinate synthetase (mitochondria)	70 min	(13)
Alanine-aminotransferase (soluble)	0.7–1.0 day	(15)
Catalase (peroxisomal)	1.4 day	(14)
Tyrosine aminotransferase (soluble	1.5 hr	(16)
Tryptophan oxygenase (soluble)	2 hr	(17)
Glucokinase (soluble)	1.25 day	(18)
Arginase (soluble)	4–5 day	(9)
Glutamic-alanine transaminase	2–3 day	(19)
Lactate dehydrogenase isozyme-5	16 day	(20)
Cytochrome c reductase (endoplasmic reticulum)	60–80 hr	(21)
Cytochrome b_5 (endoplasmic reticulum)	100–200 hr	(21)
NAD glycohydrolase (endoplasmic reticulum)	16 day	(22)
Hydroxymethylglutaryl CoA reductase (endoplasmic reticulum)	2–3 hr	(23
Acetyl CoA carboxylase (soluble)	2 day	(24)
Cell fractions		
Nuclear	5.1 day	(25)
Supernatant	5.1 day	(25)
Endoplasmic reticulum	2.1 day	(25)
Plasma membrane	2.1 day	(25)
Ribosomes	5.0 day	(26)
Mitochondria	4–5 day	(15)

SUBSTRATE

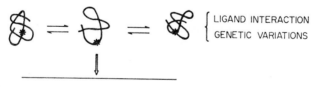

DEGRADING SYSTEM

NONSPECIFIC PROTEASE-PEPTIDASE

SPECIFIC INACTIVATING PROTEIN

LYSOSOME

LIGAND INTERACTION
GENETIC VARIATIONS

INHIBITION
  aa or aa-sRNA

ACTIVATION

SYNTHESIS

Figure 4. Summary of possible means of regulating protein degradation.

metabolic intermediates, and other proteins. The importance of ligand interaction has been well documented in protecting or labilizing proteins to a variety of physical and enzymatic inactivations. The importance of ligand interaction is suggested by the studies of Litwack & Rosenfield (33) showing a good correlation between in vivo turnover of several pyridoxal-containing enzymes and their affinity for pyridoxal phosphate. In addition, Katanuma and his group (see this volume) have shown that ornithine transaminase is subjected to specific proteolysis only in the apo- form. These results suggest that for these enzymes, the first step leading to degradation is dissociation of the cofactor.

The model that emerges, then, is one in which protein molecules are individually available to a degradative process which is present at all times. Shifting concentrations of substrates, cofactors, etc., as occurs under various metabolic and growth conditions, would lead to a variety of effects on specific enzyme, either to stabilize or labilize them. Such a concept has been expressed by Grisolia (34) and Pine (6). Also consistent with this model is the finding that there is a correlation between rates of turnover of total protein and their susceptibility to degradation by trypsin and pronase (Fig. 2). The importance of the conformation of the protein in determining rates of turnover has been demonstrated also in bacteria. Goldberg (35) has shown that protein degradation is accelerated when amino acid analogs are incorporated into proteins of E. coli, either as studied in vivo, or as degraded in extracts by exogeneous proteases. Further support comes from studies of Goldschmidt (36) showing that specific mutations in regions of the β-galactosidase gene result in a protein that is extremely rapidly degraded by endopeptidase attack.

Such a concept would also explain the development of heterogeneity of rate constants of degradation. Thus, one can readily envisage evolutionary pressure for the retention of those mutations that either increase or decrease stability of a protein, depending on whether rapid or slow turnover is advantageous to the organism for a specific protein.

2. <u>Alterations</u> <u>in</u> <u>activity</u> <u>of</u> <u>a</u> <u>degradative</u> process. Obviously the rate of degradation may also be
dependent on the activity of the degrading system, as
controlled by activation-inhibition, translocation
within a cell, or de novo synthesis of degrading enzymes. Considerations of enzymatic mechanisms are
hampered by lack of suitable mutants in the degradative process itself. Although a considerable amount
of effort has been expended in attempted isolation of
turnover mutants in bacteria (Goldberg, Bukhari, &
Chang, this volume), no such mutants have been obtained.
It is likely that this results from the existence of a
number of proteases, any one of which can effect degradation of proteins. Another problem involves the
identification of the products of specific protein
degradation once a protein has lost enzymatic activity
or immunologic reactivity. In addition, there are
several curious observations that must be taken into
account in formulation of suitable mechanism(s) for
degradation. Thus, in both animal and bacterial systems, inhibition of energy production and protein synthesis inhibits protein degradation (37). Various
explanations have been offered for such observations,
including cofactor requirements, necessity for maintaining structural or metabolic integrity of organelles,
and requirement for continued synthesis of degradative
enzymes that are turning over rapidly. More indirect,
but equally plausible from the experimental data available, are effects of accumulated amino acids, tRNA
species, alterations in cofactor levels, etc., which
may regulate by ligand interaction the activity of
degradative enzymes, or the conformation of proteins
as substrates for the degradative process.

One obvious candidate for a degradative system is
the lysosome, which occurs in virtually all cells (38).
Lysosomes are intracellular organelles that contain
acid hydrolases and are currently envisaged to be involved in the autophagy of discrete areas of cytoplasm. It is most difficult to conceive that lysosomes are involved in that protein degradation whose
properties involve randomness and heterogeneity of

degradation-rate constants among different proteins, whether so-called "soluble" proteins or those associated with membranes. Thus, some mechanism would be required for the recognition of whether a protein molecule were to be degraded, perhaps involving transport into a lysosome, acetylation, formylation, deamination (3), or limited proteolysis, followed by lysosomal engulfment. To this writer, it seems reasonable to propose that the system of lysosomes is important where cell involution or gross changes in rates of protein degradation occur, such as starvation and cell death, whereas the degradation that occurs in normal steady-state conditions involves a system(s) not clearly understood at present. This could involve lysosomes, but acting as a sieve, rather than in an "all-or-none" fashion.

Another possibility is that there are specific degrading enzymes for specific proteins. Most notable of this type of mechanism are the studies of Katanuma and his colleagues (this volume) on the existence of a so-called "group specific" protease that carried out limited cleavage of pyridoxal-containing enzymes, but only in the apo- form. The level of this enzyme is also regulated, and is elevated in animals on a pyridoxal-deficient diet.

At one extreme, then, we might propose that the degradation of each protein requires a specific protein. This, however, is impossible since the continual replacement of essentially all proteins would require that there exist a protein to degrade a protein..... ad infinitum. It is most likely that, just as there are also a number of different enzymes that hydrolyze RNA in an organism such as E. coli, there are also a number of different types of proteases in animal cells (39), the sum total of which results in continual protein degradation.

References

1. Schoenheimer, R. "The Dynamic State of Body Constituents", Harvard Univ. Press, Cambridge, Mass., (1942).

2. Schimke, R. T. & Doyle, D. J.   Ann. Rev. Biochem. 39, 929 (1970).
3. Hogness, D. S., Cohn, M. & Monod, J.   Biochim. Biophys. Acta 16, 99 (1955).
4. Koch, A. L. & Levy, H. R.   J. Biol. Chem. 217, 947 (1955).
5. Mandelstam, J.   Biochem. J. 69, 110 (1958).
6. Pine, M. J.   J. Bacteriol. 92, 847 (1966).
7. Swick, R. W.   J. Biol. Chem. 231, 751 (1957).
8. Buchanan, D. L.   Arch. Biochem. Biophys. 94, 500 (1961).
9. Schimke, R. T.   J. Biol. Chem. 239, 3808 (1964).
10. Swick, R. W., Koch, A. L. & Handa, D. T.   Arch. Biochem. 63, 226 (1956).
11. MacDonald, R. A.   Arch. Intern. Med. 107, 335 (1961).
12. Russell, D. & Snyder, S. H.   Proc. Nat. Acad. Sci. USA 60, 1420 (1968).
13. Marver, H. S., Collins, A., Tschudy, D. P. & Rechcigl, M., Jr.   J. Biol. Chem. 241, 4323 (1966).
14. Price, V. E., Sterling, W. R., Tarantola, V. A., Hartley, R. W., Jr. & Rechcigl, M., Jr.   J. Biol. Chem. 237, 3468 (1962).
15. Swick, R. W., Rexroth, A. K. & Stange, J. L.   J. Biol. Chem. 243, 3581 (1968).
16. Kenney, F. T.   Science 156, 525 (1967).
17. Schimke, R. T., Sweeney, E. W. & Berlin, C. M.   J. Biol. Chem. 240, 322 (1965).
18. Niemeyer, H.   Natl. Cancer Inst. Monograph 27, 29 (1966).
19. Segal, H. L. & Kim, Y. S.   Proc. Natl. Acad. Sci. USA 50, 912 (1963).
20. Fritz, P. J., White, E. L., Vesell, E. S. & Pruitt, K. M.   Proc. Natl. Acad. Sci. USA 62, 558, 1969.
21. Kuriyama, T., Omura, T., Siekevitz, P. & Palade, G. E.   J. Biol. Chem. 244, 2017 (1969).
22. Bock, K. W., Siekevitz, P. & Palade, G. E.   J. Biol. Chem. 246, 188 (1971).

23. Higgins, M., Kawachi, T. & Rudney, H.   Biochem.
      Biophys. Res. Commun. 45, 138 (1971).
24. Majerus, P. W. & Kilburn, E.   J. Biol. Chem. 244,
      6254 (1969).
25. Arias, I. M., Doyle, D. & Schimke, R. T.   J.
      Biol. Chem. 244, 3303 (1969).
26. Hirsch, C. A. & Hiatt, H. H.   J. Biol. Chem. 241,
      5936 (1966).
27. Dehlinger, P. J. & Schimke, R. T.   Biochem.
      Biophys. Res. Commun. 40, 1473 (1970).
28. Dice, J. F. & Schimke, R. T.   Arch. Biochem.
      Biophys. 158, 97 (1973).
29. Dehlinger, P. J. & Schimke, R. T.   J. Biol. Chem.
      246, 2574 (1971).
30. Dice, J. F., Dehlinger, P. J. & Schimke, R. T.
      J. Biol. Chem. 248, 4220 (1973).
31. Tweto, J., Dehlinger, P. J. & Larrabee, A. R.
      Biochem. Biophys. Res. Commun. 48, 1371 (1972).
32. Dice, J. F. & Goldberg, A. L.   Ann. Rev. Biochem.
      to be published.
33. Litwack, G. & Rosenfield, S.   Biochem. Biophys.
      Res. Commun. 52, 181 (1973).
34. Grisolia, S.   Physiol. Rev. 44, 657 (1964).
35. Goldberg, A. L.   Proc. Nat. Acad. Sci. 69, 422
      (1972).
36. Goldschmidt, R.   Nature New Biology 238, 1151
      (1970).
37. Schimke, R. T.   in "Mammalian Protein Metabolism"
      4, 177 (1970).
38. deDuve, C. & Baudhuin, P.   Physiol. Rev. 46,
      323 (1966).
39. Hartley, B. S.   Ann. Rev. Biochem. 29, 45 (1960).

INITIATING MECHANISMS OF INTRACELLULAR ENZYME DEGRADATION AND NEW SPECIAL PROTEASES IN VARIOUS ORGANS

Nobuhiko Katunuma, Eiki Kominami, Keiko Kobayashi,
Yoshitaka Hamaguchi, Yoshiko Banno, Kenji Chichibu,
Tsunehiko Katsunuma and Taiichi Shiotani

Department of Enzyme Chemistry
Institute for Enzyme Research
School of Medicine, Tokushima University
Tokushima, Japan

There is evidence that half-lives of pyridoxal enzymes were prolonged by administration of their coenzyme in vivo, especially in the B_6 deficient animal
(1). In these studies, pyridoxal enzymes were prelabeled in vivo and the effect of administration of
B_6 derivatives on degradation of the labeled enzyme
was investigated. Furthermore, using pulse labeling
technique, the in vivo incorporation of C^{14} or H^3
amino acids into the enzyme protein was performed to
determine the rate of enzyme protein synthesis. B_6
administration did not result in significant increase
in incorporation of labeled amino acid into the relevant enzyme protein. Therefore, these results suggest that the increase of pyridoxal enzyme caused by
B_6 administration is due to ability of coenzyme to
protect against degradation of B_6 enzymes rather than
due to the increased rate of synthesis. The regulation of intracellular apo-enzyme levels by coenzyme
stabilization against degradation has been proposed
previously. However, little knowledge is available
on the mechanisms of intracellular enzyme protein
degradation. Namely, what kinds of proteases parti-
cipate in the degradation of an enzyme protein? What
is the protease which acts on the initial step of the

enzyme degradation. What states of conformations of enzymes are susceptible to the protease? What is the trigger reaction for enzyme degradation in physiological conditions?

With regard to these questions, several new proteases have been demonstrated in our laboratory in various organs of rats which exhibit the desired substrate specificity for pyridoxal enzymes and which show a limited proteolysis (4,5,6). We propose that these proteases play the initiating role of intracellular enzyme degradation.

We will discuss them with respect to initial steps of intracellular enzyme degradation, and emphasize the importance of conformation states of substrate enzymes which are interconvertible between a non-susceptible and a susceptible form to specify a protease carrying out limited proteolysis.

Proteases Which Participate in Intracellular Enzyme Degradation

Proteases participating in intracellular enzyme degradation in physiological protein turnover have heretofore not been identified. Such proteases should possess the following characteristics: they are active in the neutral or weak alkaline range; they have a mode of action of limited proteolysis; they exhibit relative specificity for certain groups of enzymes; the activity or amount is regulatable under various physiological conditions.

A proteolytic activity capable of inactivating several pyridoxal enzymes has been detected in various organs of rat and highly purified from heavy mitochondrial fractions in our laboratory. The proteases located in liver, muscle, muscle layer and mucosa layer of intesting possess many common properties, but they appear to differ from each other in molecular weight and electric charge.

Protease activities were assayed as follows: apoenzyme (substrate) and suitable amounts of the protease were incubated and then after a 10-15 fold dilution with cold buffer the remaining activity of substrate

TABLE I.

Comparison of Group Specific Protease in Various Organs

Properties	Skeletal Muscle	Liver	Intestine Muscle Layer	Intestine Mucous Layer
Common Properties				
1. Substrate specificity for pyridoxal enzymes	High	High	High	High
2. Susceptibility to trypsin substrate (TAME)	No	No	No	No
3. Susceptibility to chymotrypsin substrate (ATEE)	30%	20%	1000%	25%
4. Inhibition by synthetic chymotrypsin inhibitor	No	No	No	No
5. Optimum pH in alkaline	9.0	8.6	9.0	8.6
6. Coenzyme protection (by PALP, PAMP)	Exists	Exists	Exists	Exists
7. SH inhibitor	No effect	No effect	No effect	No effect
8. Histidine modification (photo-oxidation)			No activity	
9. Tyrosine modification			No activity	
10. Modification of seryl-OH	Inhibited	Inhibited	Inhibited	Inhibited
Different Properties				
1. Molecular weight	12,000–14,000	14,000–17,000	25,000	30,000
2. Elution from DE-52 column	0.05M	0.75M (after protamine treatment 0.1M)	0.005M	0.25M
3. Reaction with antibody for GSP from intestine (muscle layer)*	–	–	+	–
4. Susceptibility to TEE*	0	0	100%	0
5. Catalytic speed	Very fast	Fast	Very slow	Very fast
6. Effect by Ca^{2+}	Inhibited	No effect	No effect	

* 100% represents OTA as a substrate.

TABLE II.

Substrate Specificity of Intracellular Proteases

Substrate	Source	Liver	Small Intestine Muscle	Small Intestine Mucosa	Skeletal Muscle
Ornithine transaminase	Rat liver	100*	100	100	100
Serine dehydratase	Rat liver	72	19	10	56
Homoserine deaminase	Rat liver	63	59	89	74
Phosphorylase	Rabbit muscle	27	22	70	108
δ-Aminolevulinic acid synthetase	Rabbit reticulocyte	6	9	–	+
Aspartate transaminase (s,m)	Rat liver	0	0	–	0
Tyrosine transaminase	Rat liver	0	0	–	0
Malate dehydrogenase	Rat kidney	0	0	0	0
Glutamate dehydrogenase	Bovine liver	0	0	0	0
Glyceraldehyde-3-phosphate dehydrogenase	Rabbit muscle	7	2	–	3
Glucose-6-phosphate dehydrogenase	Rat liver	3	–	–	–
Arginase	Rat liver	0	0	0	0
Glutaminase	Rat kidney	0	0	0	0
Pyruvate kinase (M type)	Rabbit muscle	0	0	0	0
Ornithine transcarbamylase	Rat liver	0	0	19	0
Xanthine oxidase	Rat liver	0	0	0	0
D-amino acid oxidase	Rat kidney	–	0	–	–

*Expressed as percent inactivation under specific conditions.

enzyme was assayed. Outline of the purification steps for four kinds of proteases located in different organs were similar, but solubilization methods from membrane, elution patterns on ion exchange chromatography, elution position on Sephadex column chromatography and mobility of electrophoresis differed. There are some steps in which marked increases in total activity are observed during the purification of all of the proteases. This may be related to the presence of specific inhibitors. The protease in muscle layer of intestine was crystallized and the proteases from skeletal muscle and liver are almost homogeneous judging from acrylamide gel electrophoresis. Properties of the different proteases are summarized in Table I.

On Ouchterlony double diffusion plates, antibody against crystalline muscle layer protease of intestine does not react with proteases from liver, skeletal muscle, mucosa layer of intestine, lysosomal protease (sonicated lysosome), trypsin and chymotrypsin. Furthermore, almost no inactivation of apo-ornithine transaminase was observed at pH 8.0 when incubated with disrupted lysosomal preparations. Many other properties of the proteases are different from lysosomal proteases (cathepsins) (7): (1) molecular weights are smaller than cathepsins; (2) these proteases have an optimum pH in an alkaline range, whereas lysosomal proteases have an optimum pH on the acidic side; (3) the proteases are seryl-protease but most cathepsins are thiol-proteases; (4) our proteases are localized in the heavy mitochondrial membrane. An interesting property of these proteases is the fact that they show a relative substrate specificity for the pyridoxal enzyme group as shown in Table II.

Enzymes belonging to pyridoxal enzyme group include many enzymes which are easy to degrade only in the apo-form. Apo forms of tyrosine transaminase and aspartate transaminase were difficult to inactivate by the protease, although they are pyridoxal enzymes. Electrophoretic mobility indicates that the proteases are basic proteins. Amino acid composition of muscle layer protease of intestine has rather high concentration of basic amino acid residues. The results of chemical

TABLE III

Chemical Modification of the Protease from Intestinal Muscle

Residues	Modifying Reagents	Enzyme Activities
Serine	DFP	↓
Histidine	Photooxidation (methylene blue)	↓
	TPCK	→
	TLCK	→
Tyrosine	Tetranitromethane	↓
	N-Acetylimidazole	→
Cysteine	PCMB	→
Carboxyl group	1-Ethyl-3(3-dimethylaminopropyl) carbodiimide	→
Amino group	Acetic anhydride	→

TABLE IV

REOATION BETWEEN CONFORMATION AND SUSCEPTIBILITY TO THE PROTEASE

	Method	Holo-OTA	Apo-OTA II	Product A	Product B
	10% TCA	Insoluble	Insoluble	Insoluble	Soluble
Molecular conformation	Analysis by UCA, Sephadex, gel electrophoresis (SDS)	Tetramer	Dimer	Dimer	Oligopeptide
	Molecular weight	140,000	67,000	≒ 67,000	10,000
Reaction with Anti-Holo OTA	Ouchterlony method	Bindable	Bindable	Bindable	
	Bindability	Bindable	Bindable	Bindable	
	Maximum absorption	420 mμ	420 mμ	420 mμ	
Effect of PALP addition	420 mμ/280 mμ	1/10	1/10	1/10	
	Km for PALP	10^{-6} M	10^{-6} M	10^{-6} M	
	Polymerization	Tetramer	Tetramerization	Dimer	
	OTA activity	Exists	Appears	No activity	
Amino-terminal	Dansyl chloride method	Met. or Try.	Met. or Try.	Gly.	Met. or Try.
Exposed -SH	DTNB titration	1.5/Dimer	3/Dimer	3/Dimer	
-Try	Differential spectra	3/Dimer	7/Dimer	7/Dimer	
-Try	Differential spectra	5-6/Dimer	11-12/Dimer	9-13/Dimer	
Susceptibility to group specific protease		No	Yes	No	

modifications of these proteases have indicated that
serine, histidine and tyrosine residues are involved
in enzyme catalysis (Table III).

Modifications of sulfhydryl groups, amino residues
and carboxyl residues are without effects. In studies
on the active center of a typical seryl protease group,
seryl-OH and histidyl labile protons play a role in
peptide bond hydrolysis and tyrosine or aspartate have
a role in determining specificity. Chemical modification studies do not necessarily indicate modification
of the active center of the protease, but rather alteration of the activity by steric hindrance of the protein.

Initiating Mechanisms of Degradation

The previous studies of Schimke et al. have shown
that the rate of degradation of a given protein within
a cell was heterogenous and that the rate could be
controlled by dietary, genetic hormonal conditions (11).
Schimke (12) and Segal (13) have suggested that the
degradative process of proteins does not constitute a
uniform system (lysosome) and that another system will
be required for variability in relative turnover rates
of individual enzyme proteins. Recently, Schimke et
al. have obtained evidence that protein degradation
in vivo may occur in a stepwise manner (14). If so,
proteases which degrade native enzyme proteins by
catalyzing very limited proteolysis and thereby producing relatively large fragments that are ultimately
broken down completely by other proteases, must be
considered. The specific proteases described in this
paper would seem appropriate for such a process, as
those proteases which act in the initiating step of
pyridoxal enzyme degradation. Then, the following
question will arise: what is the true trigger mechanism for intracellular enzyme degradation in the
physiological condition? We propose that the conformation of substrate (protein) is most important. Two
different kinds of conformations of the enzyme exist
in the cell and reversible conversion from a non-susceptible form to a form susceptible to an initiating

protease is necessary. We propose that a group specific protease acts on the susceptible form in the
limited proteolytic manner. The products having large
molecular weight are successively degraded into amino
acids by non-specific proteases. The alteration in
conformation of substrate enzymes which could be affected by interactions with ligands including substrate,
coenzyme, metal ion, phosphorylation or adenylation,
etc. are suggested to be important as the starting
mechanism of the degradation reactions.

Changes of susceptibility of substrate enzymes.
When animals were maintained on a vitamin B_6 deficient
diet, the total amount of pyridoxal enzymes decrease,
but the apo-enzyme proportion increases (15). The
decrease in these enzyme levels could be reversed within several hours after injection of a low dose of vitamin B_6 derivatives (6). In contrast, the levels of
non-B_6 dependent enzymes were unaffected by the treatments. The results suggest that the increase in pyridoxal enzyme activities caused by B_6 administration
could be due to the ability of pyridoxal phosphate
(coenzyme) to protect this enzyme from its degradation,
and not due to increased synthesis.

Relationship between conformation change accompanied
with interconversion of holo- and apo-forms of ornithine transaminase and susceptibility of these two
forms to the protease were studied. Conformational
states of substrate enzymes relate with substrate specificity, susceptibility, and limited proteolysis mode
of proteases. It is significant that the addition of
coenzyme (pyridoxal phosphate or pyridoxamine phosphate)
protected against the inactivation of these substrates
enzymes by the protease but pyridoxine phosphate or
pyridoxamine had no protective effect. It might be
that it is necessary to keep the binding site for the
coenzymes vacant when pyridoxal enzymes are subjected
to inactivation. This may suggest that the susceptibility of the substrate may depend upon the differences
in tertiary structure of apo and holo-forms of the substrate protein. The relationship between the conformations of holo form, apo form, and product and susceptibility to the protease are compared in Table IV.

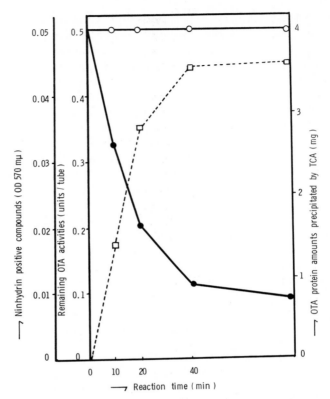

Figure 1:   Relationship between inactivation of
ornithine transaminase and breakdown of its protein
by the group specific protease from skeletal
muscle.   Each reaction mixture contained 4 mg
of apo-ornithine transaminase, 6.3 units of group
specific protease and 200 μmoles potassium phosphate buffer, pH 8.5, in a final volume of 1.0 ml.
After incubation for 0, 10, 20, 40 and 80 minutes
remaining activity of ornithine transaminase (●),
TCA precipitable protein (0) and the amount of
ninhydrin positive material in the TCA soluble
fraction (□) were determined.

Differences in the protein structure between holo-ornithine transaminase and apo-ornithine transaminase (Peak II) include subunit numbers (degree of polymerization), and the number of exposed -SH, tyrosine and tryptophan residues.

There are two forms of apo-ornithine transaminase; one is a tetramer (Peak I) and the other is dimer (Peak II) and the both forms are susceptible. Therefore, the degree of polymerization may not be so important to the susceptibility. Rather, we propose that it is necessary to keep vacant the neighbor of the binding site of coenzyme for attack by the proteases. The results using ornithine transaminase and muscle phosphorylase a (16) as the substrate suggests that the point of hydrolysis occurs near the binding site of coenzyme.

Mechanisms of limited proteolysis. The fact that the purified proteases show relative specificity for the pyridoxal enzyme group, and that their activity is very low in the holo-enzyme, suggests that they attack selected sites on the protein which binds co-enzymes. Figure 1 shows the inactivation of apo-ornithine transaminase by the purified enzyme from skeletal muscle. A reciprocal relationship exists between the decrease in transaminase activity and increase in acid-soluble, ninhydrin-reactive material. On the other hand, there was no detectable decrease in the total amount of transaminase protein precipitated by 5% trichloroacetic acid in final concentration, even after the transaminase activity was lost completely. The quantity of ninhydrin-positive substance liberated was very small, and only a few peptides were released, as detected by paper chromatography.

These results suggest that the inactivating reaction is associated with very limited proteolytic modification. The inactivated reaction products were analyzed by Sephadex column filtration and the results indicate that inactivated precipitable protein (Product A) is similar in molecular weight to the original enzyme protein, and that one polypeptide (Product B) is liberated.

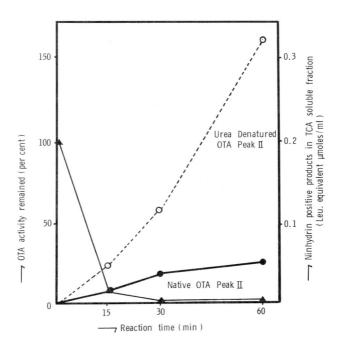

Figure 2: Susceptibility of native and urea-
denatured ornithine transaminase to group specific
protease. Urea denatured enzyme was obtained by
treatment of enzyme at 25° for 30 min in the presence of 8M urea, followed by passage through
Sephadex G-25 column chromatography equilibrated
with 0.05M potassium phosphate buffer, pH 8.0.
Reaction mixtures containing 1.4 mg enzyme and
30 units of crystalline protease from small
intestine in a final volume of 0.75 ml (pH 8.0)
were incubated at 37° for 15, 30 and 60 min. The
reaction was stopped by addition of 0.25 ml of
25% TCA. Centrifuged supernatant was used for
assay of ninhydrin reactive material.

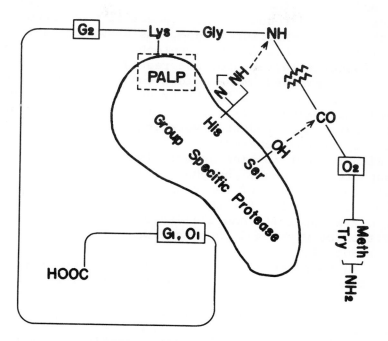

Figure 3: Hypothetical scheme of limited proteolysis of ornithine transaminase.

Analysis of the amino-terminal of apo-ornithine transaminase, Product A and Product B, were studied by the dancyl chloride method. As shown in Table IV, N-terminal, methionine or tryptophan disappeared in the Product A (after protease reaction) and new amino-terminal, branched amino acids (valine or leucine or iso-leucine) appeared in the Product A. On Ouchterlony double diffusion analysis, apo-ornithine transaminase, holo-enzyme and Product A were indistinguishable against antibody to holo-enzyme.

With respect to binding ability with pyridoxal phosphate, pyridoxal phosphate molecules per dimer unit (co-efficient of spectrum 420 mμ/280 mμ) and K_m value were similar for the apo-enzyme and Product A, but enzyme activity and ability of polymerization by addition of pyridoxal phosphate was lost completely in Product A.

As illustrated in Fig. 2, limited proteolysis could be demonstrated with native apo-ornithine transaminase as the substrate and no further degradation of Product A were observed. On the other hand, apo-ornithine transaminase denatured in 8M urea showed a random proteolysis by protease. The most essential items to show the substrate specificity, limited proteolysis and changing of susceptibility are the tertiary structure of substrate protein, especially that of neighboring coenzyme binding site.

Our hypothesis on limited proteolysis of ornithine transaminase by our proteases at the present step was offered as Fig. 3.

Regulation of group specific protease activity.
Activities which inactivate the apo forms of pyridoxal enzymes could be detected in various organs and they showed quite wide varieties in their activities. The marked increases in total activity in some steps of purification are observed with all of the proteases located in various organs, and this might be related to the existence of inhibitors in given tissues. Holzer et al. reported similar proteases in yeast (17) and also indicated the presence of specific protein inhibitors (18,19). It is possible that the regulator of the specific protease activities by alterations of

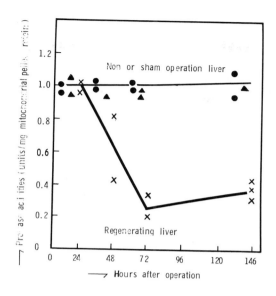

Figure 4: Changes of group specific protease
activity in regenerating liver. Partial hepatectomy was performed according to the method of
Higgins & Anderson (21). At hours indicated
after operation, 10% mitochondrial suspensions
(w/v) were prepared with pH 7.5, 0.05M potassium
phosphate buffer and sonicated. The precipitates
of sonicated mitochondrial suspension were collected by centrifugation at 10,000 g and were
suspended with pH 8.5, 0.5M potassium phosphate
buffer to 10% suspension. The protease activities
were assayed according to the method of Katunuma
et al. (7).

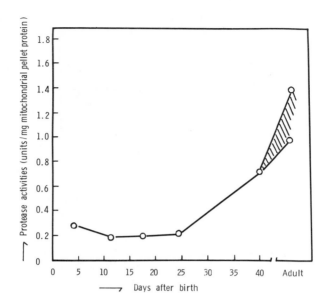

Figure 5: Changes of the liver protease during development. The precipitates of mitochondrial suspensions (0.5M potassium phosphate buffer, pH 8.5) were collected by the same method as in Fig. 4. The protease activities were assayed according to the method of Katunuma et al. (7).

inhibitor concentrations also occurs in animal systems.

It is well known that many pyridoxal enzymes in liver are responsive to several physiological states, including dietary, hormonal, or nerve alterations (20). Regenerating liver and neonatal liver shows very low protease activity. The changes of protease activities in regenerating liver is shown in Fig. 4. Two days after partial hepatectomy, marked decreases of the protease activity were observed. Figure 5 shows the changes of the protease activity during development. Protease activity in the neonatal period (within two weeks) is very low and then increases rapidly to the adult level. We speculate that there may be a relationship between the appearance of protease activity and cell division cycle.

Alterations of the levels of the protease activity were also observed under various dietary conditions. Activity in skeletal muscle of rats fed on ordinary laboratory chow is considerably lower than that in skeletal muscles or starved animals or animals fed on non-protein diet. The enhancement of group specific protease activity in response to starvation or non-protein diet is consistent with the well-known fact that under these conditions there is an increase in the amount of amino acids released and transported from muscle into the blood.

A physiological role of the group specific protease in the breakdown of muscle protein is further indicated by the observation that there is a significant increase in the level of this enzyme during atrophy of the gastrocnemium muscle caused by resection of the ischial nerve. This was performed by an experiment in which only one nerve was resected at the level of the foramen infrapiriforme. Fifteen days after the operation, the muscle weight of the gastrocnemius muscle on the resected side was reduced to 50% of that of the normal side, but the level of group specific protease on the amputated side was 3 times higher than that on the normal side (6). It is also worthy to note that resection of the ischial nerve leads to a marked decrease in the level of muscle phosphorylase activity.

201

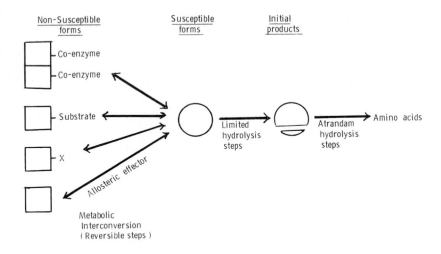

Figure 6: General process of intracellular enzyme degradation.

General Process of Intracellular Enzyme Degradation

In conclusion, we propose an hypothesis of general process of intracellular enzyme protein degradation shown in Fig. 6.

References

1. Khairallah, E. A. & Pitot, H. C. Symposium on pyridoxal enzymes (K. Yamada, N. Katunuma & H. Wada, eds.) pp. 159–164. Maruzen Co., Tokyo (1968).
2. Holten, D., Wicks, W. D. & Kenney, F. T. J. Biol. Chem. 242, 1053 (1967).
3. Greengard, O. & Gordon, M. J. Biol. Chem. 238, 3708 (1963).
4. Kominami, E., Kobayashi, K., Kominami, S. & Katunuma, N. J. Biol. Chem. 247, 6848 (1972).
5. Katunuma, N., Katsunuma, T., Kominami, E., Suzuki, K., Hamaguchi, Y., Chichibu, K., Kobayashi, K. & Shiotani, T. Advances in Enzyme Reg. (G. Weber, ed.) Vol. 11, pp. 37–51. Pergamon Press, Oxford (1973).
6. Katunuma, N. in Current Topics in Cellular Regulation (B. L. Horecker & E. R. Stadtman, eds.) Vol. 7, pp. 175–203, Academic Press, New York (1973).
7. Barrett, A. J. in Lysosomes in Biology and Pathology (J. T. Dingle & H. B. Fell, eds.) Vol. 2, pp. 245–312, North–Holland Publishing Co., Amsterdam (1969).
8. Jansen, E. F., Nutting, M. D. F. & Balls, A. K. J. Biol. Chem. 179, 189 (1949).
9. Schoellmann, G. & Shaw, E. Biochemistry 2, 252 (1963).
10. Blow, D. M., Birktoft, J. J. & Hartley, B. S. Nature 221, 337 (1969).
11. Schimke, R. T. in Current Topics in Cellular Regulation (B. L. Horecker & E. R. Stadtman, eds.) Vol. 1, pp. 77–120, Academic Press, New York (1969).

12. Schimke, R. T. in Mammalian Protein Metabolism (H. N. Munro, ed). Vol. 4, pp. 178–223, Academic Press, New York (1970).
13. Segal, H. L., Matsuzawa, T., Haider, M. & Abraham, G. J. Biochem. Biophys. Res. Commun. 36, 764 (1969).
14. Arias, I. M., Doyle, D. & Schimke, R. T. J. Biol. Chem. 244, 3303 (1969).
15. Tahami, M., Fujioka, M., Wada, H. & Taguchi, T. Proc. Soc. Exp. Biol. Med. 129, 110 (1968).
16. Matsuda, Y. & Fischer, E. H., personal communication.
17. Katsunuma, T., Schott, S. E. & Holzer, H. Eur. J. Biochem. 27, 520 (1972).
18. Ferguson, A. R., Katsunuma, T., Betz, H. & Holzer, H. Eur. J. Biochem. 32, 444 (1973).
19. Betz, H. & Holzer, H. Eur. J. Biochem., in press.
20. Knox, E. W. & Greengard, O. Advances in Enzyme Regulation (G. Weber, ed.) Vol. 3, pp. 247–313, Pergamon Press, Oxford (1965).
21. Higgins, G. M. & Anderson, R. M. Arch. Path. 12, 186 (1931).

MOLECULAR BASIS OF PROTEOLYTIC SUSCEPTIBILITY OF ORNITHINE-δ-AMINOTRANSFERASE

Takeo Matsuzawa

Department of Biochemistry
School of Medicine
Fujita-Gakuen University
Toyoake 470-11, Japan

The phenomenon of coenzyme stabilization and the rapid decrease of enzyme activity in the coenzyme deficiency state (1) has led us to the view that an apoenzyme may be labile in vivo. Several chemical modifications were carried out on the holo- and apo-ornithine-δ-aminotransferase from rat liver. Marked differences in the accessibilities of acetylation, SH titration and photo-oxidation were found (Table I). Quantitative microcomplement fixation techniques showed that the difference in accessibility of chemical modification is due to conformational changes and that such changes are completely reversible (2). These characteristics of the enzyme correlate well with susceptibility to group specific protease (3). We propose that the holoenzyme assumes a "tight state" which is stable, whereas the apoenzyme assumes a "relaxed" conformation which is labile, and is susceptible to proteolytic attack. The reversible conversion between these two distinct forms appears to be an initial critical step in the degradation process and is controlled by pyridoxal phosphate. Proteolytic susceptibility, then, is associated with a conformational state which results in exposure of substrate bond, and unmasking of an electrophylic ε-amino residue of lysine and nucleophylic SH groups in the active site. Katunuma and Sanada recently found

TABLE I.

Accessibility to Chemical Modification, Proteolytic
Susceptibility and Conformation of Ornithine-δ-Aminotransferase
in Different States (2).

	Native Holoenzyme	Apoenzyme	Apoenzyme + PALP
Number of accessible residues, per mole enzyme[1]			
Lysine[2]	0	2	0
SH group[3]	2	10 (faster)	–
Histidine[4]	6	6 (faster)	–
Conformation, complement fixation (per cent)	90	50	90
Proteolytic susceptibility	–	+	–

[1] One mole enzyme contains about 60 lysine, 22 histidine and 12 SH groups.

[2] Essential lysine residues were modified by acetylation.

[3] SH groups were titrated by 5,5'-dithiobis-(2-nitrobenzoic acid)(DTNB).

[4] 6 Histidine residues and 2 SH groups were modified by photooxidation.

further differences in availabilities of tryptophan and tyrosine residues between the holo- and apo-enzyme. In addition, we have recently found that the holoenzyme is tetramer and the apoenzyme is dimer (personal communication).

References

1. Katunuma, N. Protein Nucleic Acid Enzyme. 16, 239 (1971).
2. Matsuzawa, T. & Nishiyama, M. J. Biochem. 73, 481 (1973).
3. Katunuma, N. in Current Topics in Cellular Regulation, Vol. 7, pp. 175-203 (B. L. Horecker & E. R. Stadtman, eds), Academic Press, New York (1973).

REGULATORY DEGRADATION OF TRYPTOPHAN SYNTHASE IN YEAST

Tsunehiko Katsunuma and Helmut Holzer

Department of Enzyme Chemistry
Institute for Enzyme Research
School of Medicine
Tokushima, Japan

and

Biochemisches Institut der Universitat Freiburg
im Breisgau, Germany

It is well known that the bulk of enzymes in intact cells are degraded and therefore undergo turnover
(1,2). Recently it has become apparent that degradation by proteolytic enzymes is carefully controlled.
Katanuma et al. (3,4,5) have described "group specific
proteinases" which under certain conditions carry out
limited hydrolysis and inactivation of a limited number of enzymes.

In the present paper, our findings on tryptophan
synthase inactivating proteinases in yeast are described, and some general consequences of the role
of proteinases and their inhibitors in the regulation
of protein degradation in yeast are discussed.

In studies on factors influencing the stability of
tryptophan synthase (T-Sase) from yeast, Manney (6)
described a macromolecular factor, probably an enzyme,
which inactivated T-Sase. The activity of the inactivating system was dependent on the concentration of
vitamin and peptide mixtures in the culture medium.
On the basis of these results, Katsunuma et al (7)
and Schott & Holzer (8) have purified and characterized this principle. Two proteolyzing enzymes capable
of inactivating tryptophan synthase

(inactivase I and II) have each been purified to a single protein. Dr. Saheki in our laboratory has compared the two inactivases with proteinases A, B, and C described previously by Hata et al. (9) and Juni & Heym (10). His results indicate that inactivase I is probably identical with proteinase A and inactivase II is very similar to proteinase B. Proteinase C has no tryptophan synthase inactivating activity and therefore is omitted from the comparison. Proteinase A, B and C have been characterized with the aid of non-physiological substrates, such as albumin, casein, hemoglobin or synthetic amino acid esters not occuring in yeast.

Our findings with physiological substrates give evidence for a biological function of these proteinases. The results compiled in Table I demonstrate that inactivase I inactivates the apo- forms of T-Sase and threonine dehydratase, whereas inactivase II inactivates the apo- forms of T-Sase and aspartate aminotransferase. Neither inactivase inactivates any of three non-pyridoxal enzymes, i.e., alcohol dehydrogenase, hexokinase and glucose-6-phosphate dehydrogenase.

Concurrent with his discovery of tryptophan synthase inactivation, Manney (6) also found evidence for a macromolecular principle which prevents this inactivation. Ferguson (11) and Betz (manuscript submitted to Eur. J. Biochem.) have purified the inhibitory material. The purification procedure is summarized in Table II. Upon chromatography on QAE Sephadex, the inhibitory activity is separated into two peaks. The material from both peaks has been further purified to a homogeneous state, judging from disc electrophoresis (inhibitor I and II). The molecular weight of both inhibitors is about 10,000. Treatment with trypsin inactivates the inhibitory activity in both inhibitors. Amino acids from inhibitor II are liberated upon acid hydrolysis and about 5% carbohydrate is found with the anthrone method. Inhibitor II therefore appears to be a glycoprotein. Inhibitor II was investigated in regard to proteinase specificity.

208

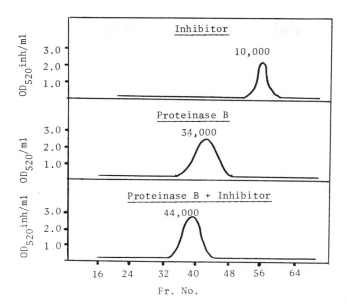

Figure 1: Filtration of proteinase B and inhibitor on Sephadex G-75. (Betz & Holzer, manuscript submitted to Eur. J. Biochem.).

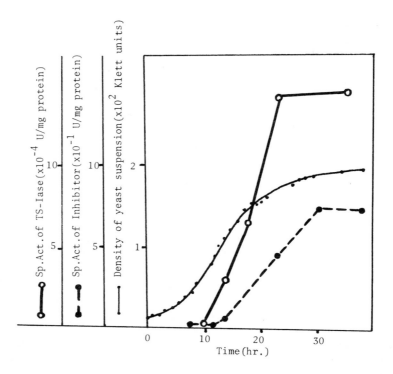

Figure 2: Dependence of the T-Sase inactivating activity and its inhibitor on the growth time. From Katsunuma, et al. (7).

TABLE II.

Purification of Yeast Inhibitors

Step	Inhibition of T-Sase inactivase activity
	Purification-fold
1. Boiled yeast extract	1
2. TCA precipitation	1.7
3. Ethanol fractionation	3.3
4. DEAE-Sephadex	15.7
5. Sephadex G-75	42.2
6. QAE-Sephadex	
Peak I	8.6
Peak II	67.3

210

Proteinases from other sources than yeast, such as trypsin, chymotrypsin and pronase are not inhibited. Of the three yeast proteinases A, B, and C, only proteinase B is inhibited by inhibitor II. The experiment presented in Fig. 1 shows that the inhibitor appears in the effluent together with proteinase B upon Sephadex gel filtration, whereas upon filtration without proteinase B, the inhibitor appears in a different fraction (Betz & Holzer, submitted Eur. J. Biochem). Therefore, the inhibition of proteinase B may be regarded as a consequence of the binding of the inhibitor to the proteinase.

Comparing the inactivating activity of yeast after growth on a minimal medium (with vitamins comprised of 0.67% Difco yeast nitrogen base and 2% glucose) and a complex medium (containing 1% Difco yeast extract, 2% Difco peptone and 2% glucose), we were able to confirm the results of Manney (6): in the yeast from a minimal medium, high T-Sase inactivating activity was observed, whereas yeast from the complex medium showed little tryptophan synthase inactivating activity. Inactivating activity in yeast grown on minimal medium was unaffected by additions of 4 or 40 mg vitamin B_6. Therefore a high B_6 content of the medium is not responsible for the low inactivating activity observed in the complex medium.

Looking for the inactivating activity and the inhibitory activity in yeast in different growth phases in the minimal medium, we found the striking phenomenon shown in Fig. 2. Whereas in the early exponential phase no inactivating activity and inhibitory activity could be detected, high inactivating activity and inhibitory activity appear at the end of the exponential phase and persist into stationary phase.

The finding supports the concept that the proteinases are concerned in mechanisms of enzyme regulation in intact cells.

References

1. Schoenheimer, R. The Dynamic State of Body
     Constituents, Harvard Univ. Press, Cambridge,
     Mass. (1942).
2. Schimke, R. T. & Doyle, D. Ann. Rev. Biochem.
     39, 929 (1970).
3. Katunuma, N., Kominami, E. & Kominami, S.
     Biochem. Biophys. Res. Commun. 45, 79 (1971).
4. Katunuma, N., Kito, K. & Kominami, E. Biochem.
     Biophys. Res. Commun. 45, 76 (1971).
5. Kominami, E., Kobayashi, K., Kominami, S. &
     Katunuma, N. J. Biol. Chem. 247, 6848 (1972).
6. Manney, T. R. J. Bacteriol. 96, 403 (1968).
7. Katsunuma, T., Schott, E., Elsasser, S. & Holzer,
     H. Eur. J. Biochem. 27, 520, (1972).
8. Schott, E. & Holzer, H. Eur. J. Biochem.,
     submitted.
9. Hata, T., Hayashi, R. & Doi, E. Agric. Biol.
     Chem. 31, 150 (1967).
10. Juni, E. & Heym, G. Arch. Biochem. Biophys. 127,
     79 (1968).
11. Ferguson, A. G., Katsunuma, T., Betz, H. & Holzer,
     H. Eur. J. Biochem. 32, 444 (1973).

PATTERN OF DEGRADATION OF SKELETAL MUSCLE GLYCOGEN PHOSPHORYLASE BY A RAT MUSCLE GROUP SPECIFIC PROTEASE

Yoshiko Matsuda and Edmond H. Fischer

Department of Biochemistry
University of Washington
Seattle, Washington 98195

When rats are fed a vitamin B_6-deficient diet, total phosphorylase content decreases by approximately 60% within 3 weeks. No apophosphorylase can be detected in skeletal muscle which, under normal conditions, contains up to 5 g of enzyme per kilogram of tissue. Phosphorylase activity also decreases markedly in animals fed a protein-free diet, or starved for one week; again, no apoenzyme can be detected. In fact, no apophosphorylase has been detected under any physiological condition. This is in contrast to the behavior of most B_6-dependent enzymes: under similar nutritional conditions, while their activities also decrease markedly, the apo/holo-enzyme ratio increases.

Two hypotheses can be suggested. First, that apophosphorylase does not exist in vivo and regulation of enzyme turnover occurs only at the level of the holoenzyme, i.e., degradation is initiated directly from the intact protein. Second, regulation occurs through degradation of apophosphorylase but this latter species is extremely susceptible to proteolysis, and therefore never accumulates in vivo to a level of detection.

A group specific protease which rapidly inactivates the apo forms of pyridoxal-P requiring enzymes has been described by Katunuma, et al. (1,2); the holoenzymes seem to be very resistant. By contrast, both the apo- and holo- forms of phosphorylase were said to be susceptible to the action of this enzyme though the mechanism of this inactivation was not investigated in detail. This report provides some information on the action pattern of the group specific protease on various forms of rabbit skeletal muscle phosphorylase and the characterization of some of the reaction products. The study was undertaken with the additional hope that it might provide a procedure to generate large fragments of phosphorylase needed for the determination of the total sequence of the enzyme presently under investigation.

The group specific protease (GSP) was prepared according to Katunuma (2) starting from an acetone powder of rat skeletal muscle; the purification involves extraction at high salt concentration, ammonium sulfate fractionation, protamine sulfate precipitation and hydroxyapatite column chromatography. The purified enzyme gives a single band on sodium dodecyl sulfate (SDS) polyacrylamide gel electrophoresis. Rabbit muscle glycogen phosphorylase was prepared according to Fischer and Krebs (3); ^{32}P-labeled phosphorylase a was prepared from phosphorylase b using purified phosphorylase kinase, Mg^{2+} and γ-^{32}P-ATP according to DeLange et al. (4). Resolution of phosphorylase b was carried out according to Shaltiel et al. (5).

Degradation of Apophosphorylase b by Rat Skeletal Muscle Group Specific Protease. The group specific protease inactivates phosphorylase a, phosphorylase b and apophosphorylase b at relative rates of 1, 1.5 and 10, respectively, in Tris-HCl buffer, pH 8.0. Proteolysis was routinely carried out at room temperature (23°) since apophosphorylases a or b are unstable above 30°. As shown in Fig. 1, apophosphorylase b irreversibly loses half of its potential activity within ca 1 hr; however, no gross decrease of the protein band appearing on SDS polyacrylamide gel electrophoresis and corresponding to the original subunit of MW 100,000 can be seen during the first hours of proteolysis, as expected if internal peptide bonds had been split. The inactivation must, therefore, result from the release of small peptides presumably located at either end of the molecule.

214

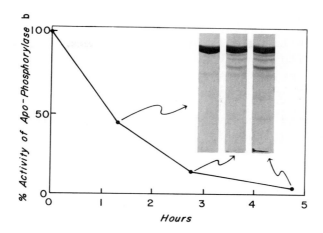

Figure 1: Degradation of apophosphorylase b by muscle
GSP. The reaction mixture contained 0.2 ml of 0.2M
Tris-HCl buffer, pH 7.5, 1 mg of apophosphorylase b
and 8 µg of GSP in a final volume of 0.5 ml; incubation was at room temperature (23°). At different
times, 50 µl aliquots were removed, and diluted with
50 µl of 50 mM mercaptoethanol containing 1 mM PMSF
and 0.2 mM pyridoxal-P; phosphorylase was assayed 15
min later. Another sample was analyzed on SDS polyacrylamide gel electrophoresis (7.5%), carried out
in 0.1M sodium phosphate buffer, pH 7.2.

Upon further proteolysis, a number of fragments with MW of ca 90,000, 85,000, 60,000, 40,000 and 30,000 are transiently produced. Two fragments (i.e., the one with MW 60,000 and, less prominently, 30,000) appear to be more resistant to further digestion and accumulate to a certain extent in the course of the reaction.

The rapid inactivation of apophosphorylase b and subsequent hydrolysis of multiple peptide bonds within the molecule is consistent with previous studies indicating that the apoenzyme has a loose structure as compared to the native protein: removal of the cofactor pyridoxal-P requires a deforming agent (such as an imidazole-citrate buffer) which distorts the molecule and exposes the cofactor assumed to be buried within a hydrophobic pocket (5). Whereas native phosphorylases a and b exist predominantly as dimers and tetramers, respectively, the apoenzyme readily dissociates to monomers particularly at higher temperatures. Nevertheless, when drastic conditions are avoided during the resolution process, both apophosphorylases b and a retain their potential catalytic activity indicating no gross or irreversible alteration in the tertiary structure of the protein. The phosphorylated site involved in the control of phosphorylase activity remains untouched since the b to a conversion proceeds readily with the apoenzyme (6). The state of aggregation of phosphorylase does not appear to affect the susceptibility of the enzyme to GSP attack: phosphorylase b and apophosphorylase b are both converted to a tetrameric species by the positive affector AMP (1 mM); yet, this nucleotide did not alter the course of the degradative process. Likewise, addition of glucose-1-P glucose-6P or glycogen was essentially without effect.

Limited Proteolysis of Holophosphorylases b and a by the Group Specific Proteases. As indicated above, and contrary to classical B_6-dependent enzymes that are highly resistant to the group specific protease as long as the cofactor is present (1,2), native phosphorylase b and a are susceptible to the action of the protease. But then, phosphorylase is an atypical B_6-requiring enzyme and the role of the cofactor has never

216

been clearly elucidated. On the one hand, pyridoxal-P has been bound in stoichiometric amounts in all phosphorylases so far investigated, and its removal leads to total inactivation. On the other hand, if the cofactor is involved in direct catalysis, it must function in a way different than that accepted for all other classical pyridoxal-P requiring enzymes, since phosphorylase reduced with NaBH$_4$ is still enzymatically active. Therefore, both a structural and catalytic role have been postulated for the cofactor (7,8), placing phosphorylase in a unique position among B$_6$-dependent enzymes even though most of the pyridoxal-P present in mammalian muscle is bound to it.

Incubation of phosphorylase b with GSP leads to the formation of two main fragments of MW 60,000 and 30,000 (Fig. 2). When gels are overloaded with reaction products, additional bands with MW 90,000 and 85,000 can be detected (not seen in Fig. 2). Proteolysis does not proceed in the presence of 1% SDS, as observed with subtilisin (9), and could be stopped by addition of this detergent.

Incubation of phosphorylase a with GSP also generates fragments of MW ca 60,000 and 30,000 but, unlike the reaction observed with phosphorylase b, no further degradation occurs within 10 hr at 30°, pH 8, as illustrated in Fig. 3. While the two large fragments could be well separated by SDS polyacrylamide gel electrophoresis, they had a strong tendency to precipitate in aqueous buffers. Therefore, the digestion products were reduced and alkylated with iodoacetic acid at the end of the reaction.

A number of attempts were made to separate these large fragments, in view of their obvious potential usefulness in the total sequence determination of the enzyme. Best results were obtained when the alkylated fragments were subjected to a hydroxyapatite column chromatography in the presence of SDS, as illustrated in Fig. 4; SDS polyacrylamide gel electrophoresis on collected fractions indicated reasonable homogeneity for the eluted fragments.

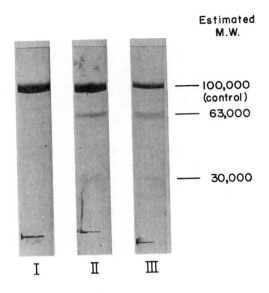

Figure 2: Degradation pattern of holophosphorylase b
by GSP on SDS polyacrylamide gel electrophoresis
contained 0.2 ml of 0.2M Tris-HCl, pH 7.5, 1 mg
of phosphorylase b, 50 μl of GSP and 1 drop of
toluene in a total volume of 0.5 ml. Incubation
was carried out at 23° for: 0 hr (I); 24 hr (II);
and 48 hr (III).

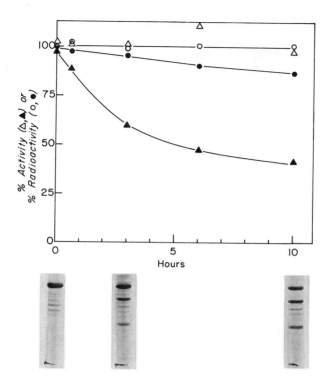

Figure 3: Degradation of holophosphorylase a by GSP.
[32]P-labeled phosphorylase a (2.5 mg) in 0.2 ml of
0.2M Tris-HCl, pH 8.0 was incubated at 30° with
10 μg of GSP in a final volume of 1.0 ml. At
various times, 50 μl of samples were removed,
diluted with PMSF and assayed for phosphorylase
activity (▲); control incubated without GSP, (△).
At the same time, 50 μl samples were added to 0.1
ml of 25 mg/ml bovine serum albumin, precipitated
with 0.8 ml of 10% trichloroacetic acid; the suspension was kept at 0° for 30 min then centrifuged.
Radioactivity was measured both in the supernatant
solution and precipitate: samples incubated with
(●) and without (○) GSP.

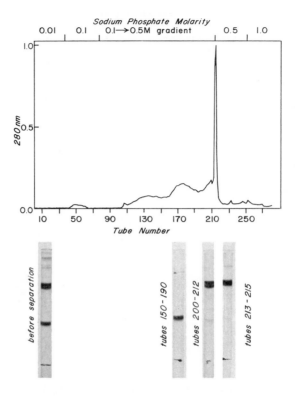

FIGURE 4: Separation of large phosphorylase peptides by
hydroxyapatite chromatography. The phosphorylase a fragments
generated by limited proteolysis were reduced with $NaBH_4$, alkylated
with ICH_2COOH and lyophylized. The residue (0.8 mg) was dissolved
in 2 ml 1% SDS, boiled for 2 min, diluted with 10 vol of 0.01 M
sodium phosphate buffer, pH 6.4, and applied to a 1.5 x 10 cm column
filled with a 1:3 (w/w) mixture of cellulose powder and Biogel HTP,
equilibrated in the same SDS (0.1%) - Na phosphate buffer. After
washing with 100 ml of buffer, elution was carried out with a
linear gradient of 0.1 to 0.5 M Na phosphate, pH 6.4, containing
0.1% SDS.

Similar limited proteolyses with separation of the reaction products were also carried out on both [^{32}P]-labeled and NaBH$_4$-reduced phosphorylases. In the first instance, very little radioactivity was released in a trichloroacetic acid-soluble form during the first 10 hr of incubation; indicating that the phosphorylated site had not been released in the form of small peptides as previously observed with tryptic or chymotryptic attacks (10,11). Essentially all the radioactivity appeared in the 30,000 MW fragment. Since the seryl residue phosphorylated in the phosphorylase b to a conversion was shown to occupy position #14 in the primary structure of the enzyme (12), the 30,000 MW fragment must originate from the amino terminal end of the molecule. This assumption is supported by the finding that it has a blocked amino terminal residue just like the native enzyme which contains an N-acetyl serine at this position.

GSP digestion of NaBH$_4$-reduced phosphorylase indicates that the covalently fixed phosphopyridoxyl residue is entirely contained in the larger, 60,000 MW fragment as determined by its characteristic fluorescence properties; this fragment contained a single isoleucyl NH$_2$-terminal residue, indicating a rather clean scission of the peptide chain.

The degradation pattern obtained with phosphorylase a described here is similar to that previously obtained by the use of subtilisin (13). At first glance, this might suggest the occurrence of points of greater susceptibility to proteolysis along the phosphorylase peptide chain. However, a totally different pattern of degradation was observed in the presence of the group specific protease isolated from the small intestine. In addition, of course, trypsin and chymotrypsin will generate an entirely different set of degradation products. Therefore, proteolysis cannot depend entirely on the structure of the protein substrate, but to a large extnt on the specificity of the protease involved. Since muscle phosphorylase nicked by GSP becomes extremely susceptible to general proteolysis, it is tempting to propose that the group specific protease initiates this degradative process in vivo.

References

1. Katunuma, N., Katsunuma, T., Lominami, E., Suzuki, K., Hamaguchi, Y., Chichibu, K., Kobayashi, K. & Shiotani, T., in Advances in Enzyme Regulation (G. Weber, ed.), Pergamon Press, Oxford, New York, Vol. 11, p. 37-51 (1973).
2. Katunuma, N., in Current Topics in Cellular Regulation (B. L. Horecker and E. R. Stadtman, eds) Academic Press, New York, Vol. 7, pp. 175-202 (1973).
3. Fischer, E. H. & Krebs, E. G. J. Biol. Chem. 231, 65 (1958).
4. DeLange, R. J., Kemp, R. G., Riley, W. D., Cooper, R. A. & Krebs, E. G. J. Biol. Chem. 243, 2200 (1968).
5. Shaltiel, S., Hedrick, J. L. & Fischer, E. H. Biochemistry 5, 2108 (1966).
6. Hedrick, J. L., Shaltiel, S. & Fischer, E. H. Biochemistry 5, 2117 (1966).
7. Fischer, E. H., Forrey, A. W., Hedrick, J. L., Hughes, R. O., Kent, A. B. & Krebs, E. G. in Chemical and Biological Aspects of Pyridoxal Catalysis (E. E. Snell, P. M. Fasella, A. Braunstein and A. Rossi Fanelli, eds.)p. 543, Pergamon Press, Oxford (1963).
8. Fischer, E. H., Kent, A. B., Sneider, E. R. & Krebs, E. G. J. Amer. Chem. Soc. 80, 2906 (1958).
9. Gounaris, A. & Ottesen, J. C. R. Tran. Lab. Carlsberg 35, 37 (1965).
10. Fischer, E. H., Graves, D. J., Snyder-Crittenden, E. R. & Krebs, E. G. J. Biol. Chem. 234, 1698 (1959).
11. Nolan, C., Novoa, W. R., Krebs, E. G. & Fischer, E. H. Biochemistry 3, 542 (1964).
12. Fischer, E. H., Cohen, P., Fosset, M., Muir, L. W. & Saari, J. C. in Metabolic Interconversion of Enzymes (Wieland, O., Helmreich, E. and Holzer, H., eds.) pp. 11-28, Springer-Verlag, Heidelberg (1972).
13. Raibaud, O. & Goldberg, M. E. Biochemistry 12, 5154 (1973).

PATHWAYS OF PROTEIN DEGRADATION. A FACTOR REGULATING HEPATIC PHOSPHOFRUCTOKINASE STABILITY

Harold L. Segal and George A. Dunaway, Jr.

Department of Biology
State University of New York
Buffalo, New York 14214

Pathways of Protein Degradation

The elucidation of the mechanism of protein degradation requires a description of the steps which lead from active protein to its constituent amino acids and their return to the metabolic pool. Of particular interest are the identification of the rate-limiting steps and the nature of the factors which regulate them. It seems likely from present knowledge that the resolution of the problem will not require the discovery of novel biochemical processes, but rather of how relatively familiar reactions are organized and integrated within the cell.

We can represent the elements of protein degradation for purposes of discussion in the following series of steps.

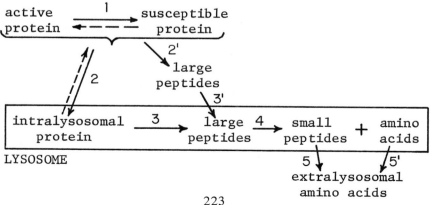

223

In step 1 we are suggesting that in many or perhaps most cases the physiologically active form of a protein may not be the one most susceptible to proteolytic attack. Coffey & deDuve have proposed in fact that denaturation is a prerequisite to proteolysis (1). While it is certainly the case that denaturation renders proteins more susceptible to proteolytic attack and that some proteins may be sufficiently labile under physiological conditions to make this process a significant one on the pathway to degradation, it is also true that a number of examples are known of proteolytic attack by cellular degradases on un-denatured proteins (2-4). These latter observations do not exclude the possibility, however, that the susceptible form is distinct from, but in equilibrium with, the physiologically active form, e.g., as a conformer (5, 6), subunit (7), or ligand-dissociated state (8). (The reverse arrow in step 1 is dashed to indicate the possibilities of both reversible and irreversible conversion to the proteolytically susceptible form.)

In step 2, we indicate a translocation of the protein to the lysosome, since present evidence indicates that the capacity of the cell to attack whole proteins resides predominantly in this organelle (9). The problem of the nature of the process by which the proteins of the cell become accessible to the lysosomal proteases is addressed by the model of deDuve & Wattiaux (10), which proposes on the basis of electron microscopic evidence that autophagic vacuoles engulf portions of cellular material, then merge with primary lysosomes containing the degradative enzymes to form the secondary lysosomes in which digestion takes place. In this process there is ample scope to account for the energy requirement for protein degradation (11). (In this regard Hayashi et al. have recently reported ATP stimulates in vitro digestion of proteins by intact but not disrupted lysosomes (12); however, it is not yet entirely clear how this observation is to be interpreted.) What is not known is whether the translocation of cell constituents into the lysosomal system is specific or random, whether the motion and merger of

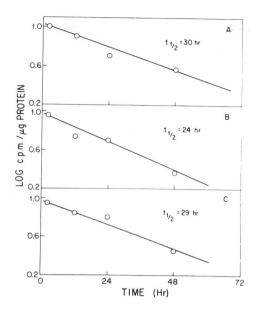

Figure 1: Half-life of total lysosomal protein and
two sub-fractions thereof. Rats were injected at
time 0 with (^{14}C)arginine labeled in the guanido
group (25 to 100 µCi/rat) and sacrificed at the
times shown thereafter. Triton WR-1339 (1 g/kg
body weight) was injected 3-1/2 days before the
scheduled time of sacrifice and the liver lysosomes isolated by the flotation method of
Leighton et al. (13). An aliquot of the resuspended lysosomal preparation was spotted onto a
filter paper disc and prepared for radioactivity
counting by the method of Mans & Novelli (14)
(graph A). The remainder of the preparation was
centrifuged and the pellet resuspended in 10 mM
acetate buffer, pH 5.0, to lyse the particles.
The soluble (graph B) and insoluble (graph C)
fractions, about equal in protein content, were
separated by centrifugation and counted. Counts
were normalized to a basis of 100 µCi injected.

vacuoles and primary lysosomes is directed, and whether
engulfed material is inevitably digested or can escape
intact, among other questions.

Step 3 (or 2', see below) represents the initial
hydrolytic step leading to inactive products and com-
mitting the protein to eventual total hydrolysis.
Since variability among proteins in rates of proteolytic susceptibility is well established, we have
relegated the specificity in degradation rates for
the most part to this step for those proteins which
enter the lysosome in an undenatured state, in order
to avoid the necessity of inventing ad hoc mechanisms
for discrimination among soluble proteins in the
ingestion step. However, to bring this model into
conformity with the principle that the rate-limiting
step in a pathway is the first irreversible one requires
that the ingestion step be considered reversible, i.e.,
that proteins once ingested may escape intact. This
proposition, largely hypothetical on the basis of
current knowledge, is represented by the dashed
reverse arrow in step 2. One condition which would
favor the possibility of a return of the lysosomal
contents to the cytosol in an intact state is a relatively rapid turnover of the lysosome itself. We have
now found that this is indeed the case (Fig. 1). The
half-life of 24-30 hrs obtained for total liver lysosomal protein and two subfractions thereof is considerably less than that of a number of discrete proteins
and organelles of this organ (15), thus requiring that
these constituents enter the lysosome more than once
on the average if the eventual initial hydrolytic step
takes place therein.

It would appear, on the basis of recent reports,
that the initial proteolytic attack cannot be univers-
ally ascribed to lysosomal proteases. Katunuma and
his associates have obtained evidence for the existence of neutral proteases, presumably non-lysosomal,
which have the capacity to split specifically the
apo forms of pyridoxal phosphate-, NAD-, and FAD-
requiring enzymes, respectively (16-18). Step 2',
representing a by-pass of the lysosome in the initial

226

proteolytic step, and would include this type of process. The initial products would presumably enter the lysosome (step 3') where further digestion would occur.

We have distinguished the initial hydrolytic split (step 3 or 2') from further hydrolysis (step 4 <u>et seq</u>.) in order to emphasize that the former, as the first unequivocally irreversible step in the overall process, is a potential site of the regulatable, rate-limiting reaction in protein degradation. Previous reports from this laboratory have in fact demonstrated the regulatability of this step in the degradation of model enzymes studied (3).

Coffey & deDuve (1) have shown that digestion of proteins by lysosomal extracts is extensive (step 4), releasing almost half the amino acids in the free state and the bulk of the remainder as dipeptides. Further hydrolysis of the peptides required the action of soluble neutral peptidases (step 5). Thus, it may be presumed that the small peptides produced in step 4 diffuse from the lysosome into the cytosol where final hydrolysis to amino acids takes place. This presumption is consistent with the findings that the lysosome is permeable to substances of molecular weight up to approximately that of dipeptides (19,20).

We have indicated an additional step (step 5') representing the translocation to the cytosol of amino acids formed in the lysosome. Two separate lines of evidence suggest that these pools are not in equilibrium. Firstly, Tappel et al. have found that the free amino acid concentration within lysosomes is as much as an order of magnitude higher than that in the remainder of the cell (21,22). Secondly, Mortimore et al. (23) have obtained evidence for a pool of amino acids which is not in equilibrium with the extracellular pool and which appears to arise from protein breakdown. These observations taken together are highly supportive of the premise that the bulk of protein breakdown in the cell takes place within the lysosome.

Within this overall pathway several sites suggest themselves as points at which the regulatable, rate-limiting step may occur in the degradation of a given protein. In the case of proteins where irreversible denaturation precedes translocation to the lysosome and/or proteolysis, the rate of step 1 determines the specific rate of protein degradation. Even if step 1 is reversible it may be rate-limiting if it is slow relative to subsequent processes. Litwack & Rosenfield have suggested that this may be the case with coenzyme associated enzymes, where they propose that cofactor dissociation produces the susceptible form (8).

The possibility of the lysosomal ingestion process (step 2) as a rate-limiting site may be considered. This could be the case if ingestion is specific. However, to be generally so would require a recognition site on the ingesting particle for each substance ingested, which is exceedingly difficult to visualize. If, on the other hand, this process is non-specific but involves an engulfment of whatever materials are in the volume segregated by vacuole formation, then it follows that the fractional rate of uptake is the same for all cell constituents. Since fractional degradation rates (i.e., the rate constant of degradation, k_d) of cell constituents are not identical, this process cannot in general be rate-limiting if it is random, except for those constituents which are relatively stable in the cytosol but are rapidly denatured and/or proteolyzed in the lysosome. All such substances would then have identical half-lives which would reflect the rate of lysosomal ingestion (24).

Step 3 is a kind of reaction where specificity of rate is thoroughly established. However, as pointed out above, for step 3 to be rate-determining requires that the previous step in the pathway (step 2) be reversible. To what degree this is the case should be accessible to further experimental investigation. Step 2' is also one where specificity is expected and would be rate-limiting except where step 1 (e.g., coenzyme dissociation) is slow. None of the succeeding steps (3',4,5, or 5') could be limiting insofar as protein removal rates are concerned, although they may be in the return of amino acids from proteins to the available pool (21-23).

228

A Factor Regulating Hepatic Phosphofructokinase Stability

Some recent results add another element to the large picture, specifically in the area of the regulation of degradation. Dunaway & Weber have recently discovered that the level of the major hepatic isozyme of phosphofructokinase, PFK-L_2, is reduced in diabetes and starvation, and have demonstrated in the case of the latter that this change is a result of an increased degradation rate of the enzyme (25,26). We can now report the existence of a labile, non-dialyzable factor in rat liver supernatant fluid which protects liver phosphofructokinase against thermal inactivation. This factor is not present in other tissues examined, except kidney, and does not affect the stability of other hepatic enzymes tested (flucokinase and pyruvate kinase). The level of the factor is decreased in starvation, where the in vivo degradation rate of phosphofructokinase is increased, and restored with refeeding. The level of factor and of phosphofructokinase also change in parallel with insulin deprivation and administration. These findings suggest that regulation of phosphofructokinase levels in the liver is mediated by alterations in the content of the protective factor.

Methods. PFK-L_2 was isolated from rats by the method of Dunaway & Weber (27) and was assayed as they describe. The final preparations were in a solution of 50 mM Tris-Cl, pH 8.0, 50 mM NaF, 10 mM dithiothreitol, and 1.0 mM ATP, and contained about 200 units/ml of specific activity 50 to 70.

Liver supernatant fluid as a source of the protective factor was obtained by homogenization of rat liver at 0° in 2 volumes of 50 mM Tris-Cl, pH 8.4, followed by centrifugation at 100,000 x g for 45 min. Low molecular weight compounds were removed by passage of 5 ml of the supernatant solution through a column (1.5 cm x 15 cm) of Sephadex G-25 (coarse) equilibrated with the homogenizing solution. A unit of protective factor is defined as the amount which extends by 1 min the half-life of PFK-L_2 during the inactivation reaction (28).

229

Table I

Tissue Distribution of PFK-L$_2$ Protective Factor

Incubations were as described in Fig. 2 with 16 mg of protein from the tissue indicated. Tissue extracts were prepared as described in the text for liver.

Tissue	Protective factor (units)
liver	31
kidney	25
brain	12
heart	11
muscle	8
serum	4
testis	4
serum albumin (bovine)	5

from Dunaway and Segal (28)

Table II

Specificity of PFK-L$_2$ Protective Factor

Incubations were as described in Fig. 2. The liver extract contained 22 mg of protein/ml.

Enzyme	Half-lives (min)	
	control	+ 2.0 ml liver extract
PFK-L$_2$ (1.25 units)	5	57
PFK-L$_2$ (2.5 units)	5	58
PFK-L$_2$ (5.0 units)	5	56
glucokinase (1.8 units)	3	3.5
pyruvate kinase L (1.2 units)	3	3

from Dunaway and Segal (28)

Table III

Lability of the Protective Factor and its Stabilization by Glucose

Incubations were as described in Fig. 2 with 1.0 ml of liver supernatant fluid (21.5 mg protein). Glucose, when added was at a concentration of 0.25 M. Glucose itself had no effect on the half-life of PFK-L$_2$.

Conditions of storage	Protective activity (% of initial[a])	
	time of storage	
	24 hr	48 hr
4°, no glucose	0	0
4°, + glucose	100	60
-20°, no glucose	10	0
-20°, + glucose	100	72
liq. N, no glucose	20	0
liq. N, + glucose	100	72

[a] The initial activity of the fresh supernatant fluid was 25 units/ml.

from Dunaway and Segal (28)

230

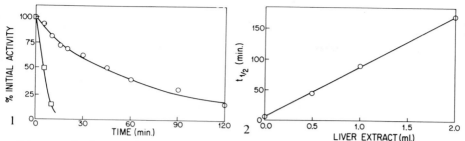

Figure 2 (left): Thermal inactivation of PFK-L$_2$.
Incubations were at 37° with 20 µl of PFK-L$_2$ solution plus 2.0 ml of homogenizing buffer (pH 8.0 at
this temperature)(squares), or 1.0 ml of homogenizing buffer plus 1.0 ml of liver supernatant fluid
(20.3 mg protein/ml) prepared as described in the
text (circles). From Dunaway & Segal (28).

Figure 3 (right): Proportionality of PFK-L$_2$ half-
life (t-1/2) to concentration of protective factor.
The experiment was carried out as in Fig. 2 with
various volumes of liver supernatant fluid (30.6
mg protein/ml) added in place of buffer. From
Dunaway & Segal (28).

Table IV

Effect on Liver Protective Factor Levels of Fasting and
Refeeding and of Diabetes and Insulin Treatment

Data are averages of 2 animals. Refeeding began after
6 days of fasting. Rats were made diabetic by the injection
(i.p.) of 200 mg alloxan monohydrate per kg body weight
after a 30 hr fast and were used 7 days later. Insulin treatment was 2 units/day (s.c.) of protamine zinc insulin
(Lilly). Blood sugar levels of the diabetic rats were between
500 and 550 mg per 100 ml. Incubations were as described
in Fig. 2 with 1.0 ml of liver supernatant fluid.

Treatment	Protective factor	DNA
	% of control[a]	mg/g liver
controls	100	1.9
3 day fast	41	3.1
6 day fast	12	4.0
1 day refeed	140	2.5
2 day refeed	79	2.1
3 day refeed	91	1.9
diabetic	26	2.8
1 day insulin	180	2.2
2 day insulin	116	1.7
3 day insulin	89	1.9

[a] The control value was 91 units/mg DNA.

from Dunaway and Segal (28)

Partially purified preparations of rat liver glucokinase and pyruvate kinase L were obtained by methods
adapted from published procedures (29,30).

Results. Figure 2 shows the time course of inactivation of PFK-L$_2$ in the absence and presence of protective factor. Proportionality of the half-time
extension to the amount of factor is demonstrated in
Fig. 3.

Table I contains the results of tests of the ability
of extracts of other rat tissues and a non-specific
protein to protect PFK-L$_2$. As can be seen only liver
and kidney possessed significant protective ability.
Table II demonstrates that the effect is independent
of PFK-L$_2$ concentration as predicted from the model
(28) and the lack of protective effect on liver glucokinase and pyruvate kinase L [the isozymes which, like
PFK-L$_2$, are the ones responsive to nutritional and
hormonal state (31,32)].

The lability of the factor and the ability of glucose to stabilize it are shown in Table III.

Table IV shows the effects on protective factor
levels of fasting and refeeding and of diabetes and
insulin treatment. With both fasting and diabetes
there was a marked reduction in protective factor
levels which was reversed by refeeding or insulin
treatment, respectively. The reversal in both cases
was rapid, overshooting normal levels on the first
day before returning to control values.

Discussion. The results presented here demonstrate
the existence of a factor in liver and kidney which
protects the major liver isozyme of phosphofructokinase (PFK-L$_2$) against thermal inactivation. This
factor appears to be a protein as indicated by its
size and lability, but this remains to be conclusively
demonstrated by isolation. The lack of protective
effect toward the other enzymes tested and the cor-
respondence in tissue distribution of the factor and
the PFK-L$_2$ isozyme (27) permit the tentative conclusion that the factor is specific for this enzyme.
This is consistent with other evidence that only the
PFK-L$_2$ isozyme is subject to regulatory control while
the minor isozyme of liver, PFK-L$_1$, is not (25,27).

The correlation between changes in the level of the protective factor and of PFK-L_2 in altered nutritional and hormonal states and the time relationships thereof suggest a close interdependency between the two. Since the decline and restoration of PFK-L_2 levels, at least in the case of fasting and refeeding, have been shown to reflect changes in the degradation rates of the enzyme (25) it can be proposed that the protective factor plays a direct role in determining the stability of the enzyme in vivo.

Acknowledgements

This work was supported by a grant from the U. S. Public Health Service (AM-08873). Mr. John A. Brown performed the experiment in Fig. 1. We thank Mr. Ronald M. Schreiber for his assistance in other of these experiments.

References

1. Coffey, J. W. & deDuve, C. J. Biol. Chem. 243, 3255 (1968).
2. Otto, V. K. & Schepers, P. Z. physiol. Chem. 348, 482 (1967).
3. Haider, M. & Segal, H. L. Arch. Biochem. Biophys. 148, 228 (1972).
4. Betz, H., Gratzl, M. & Remmer, H. Z. physiol. Chem. 354, 1 (1973).
5. Markus, G. Proc. Nat. Acad. Sci. 54, 253 (1965).
6. Taninchi, H., Moravek, L. & Anfinsen, C. B. J. Biol. Chem. 244, 460- (1969).
7. Dice, J. F., Dehlinger, P. J. & Schimke, R. T. J. Biol. Chem. 248, 4220 (1973).
8. Litwack, G. & Rosenfield, S. Biochem. Biophys. Res. Commun. 52, 181 (1973).
9. Brostrom, C. O. & Jeffay, H. J. Biol. Chem. 245, 4001 (1970).
10. deDuve, C. & Wattiaux, R. Ann. Rev. Physiol. 28, 435 (1966).
11. Steinberg, D., Vaughan, M. & Anfinsen, C. B. Science 123, 389 (1956).

12. Hayashi, M., Hiroi, Y., & Natori, Y. Nature New Biol. 242, 163 (1973).

13. Leighton, F., Poole, B., Beaufay, H., Baudhuin, P., Coffey, J. W., Fowler, S., & deDuve, C. J. Cell Biol. 37, 482 (1968).

14. Mans, R. J. & Novelli, G. D. Biochem. Biophys. Res. Commun. 3, 540 (1960).

15. Schimke, R. T. in Mammalian Protein Metabolism (H. N. Munro, ed.) Vol. IV, p. 177, Academic Press, New York (1970).

16. Katunuma, N., Kominani, E., Kominami, S., Kito, K., & Matsuzawa, T. in Metabolic Interconversion of Enzymes (O. Wieland, E. Helmreich & H. Holzer, eds.) p. 159, Springer-Verlag, Berlin (1972).

17. Katunuma, N., Kito, K., & Kominami, E. Biochem. Biophys. Res. Commun. 45, 76 (1971).

18. Kominami, E., Kobayashi, K., Kominami, S., & Katunuma, N. J. Biol. Chem. 247, 6848 (1972).

19. Ehrenreich, B. A. & Cohn, Z. A. J. Exp. Med. 129, 227 (1969).

20. Lloyd, J. B. Biochem. J. 121, 245 (1971).

21. Tappel, A. L., Shibko, S., Stein, M., & Susz, J. P. J. Food Sci. 30, 498 (1965).

22. Tappel, A. L. in Lysosomes in Biology and Pathology (J. T. Dingle & H. B. Fell, eds.) Vol. 2, p. 207, North-Holland Publishing Co. Amsterdam (1969).

23. Mortimore, G. E., Woodside, K. H., & Henry, J. E. J. Biol. Chem. 247, 2776 (1972).

24. Segal, H. L., Matsuzawa, T., Haider, M. & Abraham, G. J. Biochem. Biophys. Res. Commun. 36, 764 (1969).

25. Dunaway, G. A., Jr., & Weber, G. Arch. Biochem. Biophys. in press (1974).

26. Weber, G. (1974) (this volume).

27. Dunaway, G. A., Jr., & Weber, G. Arch. Biochem. Biophys., in press (1974).

28. Dunaway, G. A., Jr. & Segal, H. L. Biochem. Biophys. Res. Commun. 56, 689.

29. Pilkis, S. J. Arch. Biochem. Biophys. 149, 349 (1972).
30. Susor, W. A., & Rutter, W. J. Biochem. Biophys. Res. Commun. 30, 14 (1968).
31. Salas, M., Vinuela, E., & Sols, A. J. Biol. Chem. 238, 3535 (1963).
32. Tanaka, T., Harano, Y., Sue, F., & Morimura, H. J. Biochem. 62, 71 (1967).

THE EFFECT OF ATP ON PROTEIN DEGRADATION IN RAT LIVER LYSOSOMES

Yasuo Natori

Department of Nutritional Chemistry
Tokushima University School of Medicine
Tokushima, Japan

An interesting aspect of protein catabolism is its apparent energy requirement. In 1953, Simpson (1) studied the release of radioactive amino acids from proteins labeled in vivo in rat liver slices and he showed that this process was inhibited by inhibitors of energy metabolism. Simpson's finding was confirmed and extended by Steinberg & Vaughan (2) and also by Korner & Tarver (3). A more direct test for this energy requirement was performed by Penn (4) who showed that the in vitro degradation of serum albumin at neutral pH by the particulate fractions derived from liver homogenate was stimulated by added ATP. A similar finding was reported by Umaña (5). But recent studies (6,7,8,9) failed to reproduce the direct stimulatory effect of ATP in a homogenate of rat liver. Thus the present state of our knowledge on the relationship between energy and protein catabolism still remains inconclusive.

Lysosomes are known to contain cathepsins with acid pH optima and are believed to be the major site of protein degradation in vivo (10,11). We have investigated the effect of added ATP on the activities of cathepsins and a few representative lysosomal enzymes in the intact as well as disrupted lysosomes. Here we describe our results, which indicate that ATP enhances the catheptic activity in the intact lysosomes by promoting the transport of the substrate protein into the lysosomes.

237

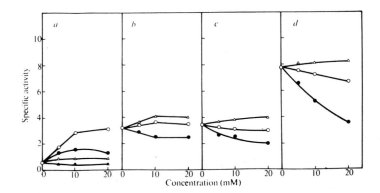

Figure 1: Effect of ATP and Mg^{2+} on the proteolytic activity of various lysosomal preparations. The intact lysosomes were disrupted by the addition of 'Triton' X-100 to a final concentration of 0.13%. The concentrations of ATP or $MgSO_4$ in the mixtures are given on the abscissa. Cathepsin was assayed by the method of Gianetto and deDuve (18) and the specific activity is expressed as units/mg of lysosomal protein, where one unit corresponds to 1 μg of tyrosine-equivalent produced per min. The lysosomal preparations used were, (a) intact, (b) 'Triton'-treated, (c) sonicated, (d) acetone-powder extract. 0, ATP plus Mg^{2+}; 0, ATP; Δ, Mg^{2+}; Δ, AMP plus Mg^{2+}.

Effect of ATP and Mg^{2+} on Proteolysis

Lysosomes were prepared from the livers of rats by the method of Sawant et al. (11) and the catheptic activity was assayed in an isotonic medium (0.25 M sucrose) at pH 4.5 using hemoglobin as a substrate. In the first place, the effect of ATP and Mg^{2+}, either singly or in equimolar combinations, on the proteolytic activity of intact lysosomes was studied. As shown in Fig. 1a, increasing concentrations of Mg^{2+} had a slight activation effect on the hydrolysis of hemoglobin. Addition of ATP to the reaction mixture caused stimulation up to 10 mM, but further increase to 20 mM was inhibitory. Addition of equimolar combinations of ATP and Mg^{2+} caused a linear increase in proteolytic activity up to 10 mM, where a plateau was reached representing 5 to 6-fold stimulation from the basal level. Addition of AMP in place of ATP caused no stimulation.

Next, the effect of ATP and Mg^{2+} on the Triton-treated or sonicated lysosomes was investigated. These treatments disrupt the membranous structure of lysosomes and cause the release of structure-confined enzymes into the reaction media. Figures 1b and 1c show that the basal levels of enzymatic activity were greatly elevated. The stimulatory effect of ATP had then disappeared and ATP became inhibitory to proteolytic activity. The addition of Mg^{2+} caused slight stimulation.

Although sonication and 'Triton'-treatment would have effectively disrupted the membranous structure of lysosomes, the lipid components of the membrane were not removed from the reaction systems. Thus, the effect of ATP and Mg^{2+} in the system of acetone-powder extract was investigated. The acetone treatment should completely destroy the lipoprotein complex which constitutes the membranous structure of lysosomes. The results with acetone-powder extract are presented in Fig. 1d. By contrast with the preceding systems, ATP clearly inhibited proteolysis. That this inhibition is not the direct inhibitory effect of ATP on the proteolytic system was indicated by the

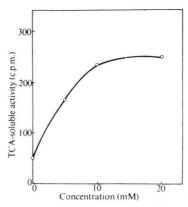

Figure 2: Effect of ATP plus Mg^{2+} on the hydrolysis
of ^{14}C-labeled proteins. ^{14}C-Labeled cytosolic
proteins (23,000 dpm) were incubated with intact
lysosomes in 0.25M sucrose, 0.05M acetate buffer
(pH 4.5). The concentrations of ATP and MgSO$_4$ in
the reaction mixtures are given on the abscissa.
After incubation for 30 min at 37°C, trichloroacetic acid-soluble radioactivity was counted.

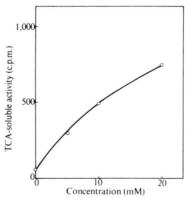

Figure 3: Effect of ATP plus Mg^{2+} on the hydrolysis
of ^{125}I-labeled proteins. ^{125}I-labeled cytosolic
proteins (17,000 cpm) were incubated with intact
lysosomes in the same manner as in Fig. 2.

240

reversal of this inhibition with the addition of an equimolar amount of Mg^{2+} to the system. Mg^{2+} alone was found to be slightly stimulatory to the system. The apparent inhibitory action of ATP in this system, then, should be due to the well-known chelating ability of ATP to remove essential Mg^{2+} from the enzyme system. We may conclude that ATP itself is neither inhibitory nor stimulatory to the proteolytic enzymes. Therefore, the effect of ATP plus Mg^{2+}, observed with intact lysosomes (Fig. 1a), does not represent the direct activation of proteolytic enzymes, but rather seems to reflect the change in the topological relationship between enzymes and substrate.

So far, the effect of ATP was tested with hemoglobin as a substrate. The next question to be answered is whether the ATP effect is specific for hemoglobin degradation or is applicable to other proteins in general. The effect of ATP plus Mg^{2+} on the degradation of rat liver cytosolic proteins by the intact lysosomes was tested. The soluble proteins of rat liver were labeled by two different methods, internal and external. The internal labeling was performed by intraperitoneal injection of ^{14}C-leucine into rats and subsequent isolation of the labeled cytosol proteins from the livers. The external labeling was performed by reacting the isolated cytosol proteins with sodium ^{125}I-iodide in the presence of 'Chloramine T'. The effect of ATP plus Mg^{2+} on the hydrolysis of internally-labeled cytosolic proteins by the intact lysosomes is shown in Fig. 2. The proteolysis was indeed dependent on ATP-Mg^{2+}, in much the same manner as in the case of hemoglobin degradation (Fig. 1a). Essentially the same result was obtained with ^{125}I-labeled proteins as substrate (Fig. 3). We conclude that the effect of ATP on the degradation of proteins by the intact lysosomes is fairly general as regards the kind of proteins used as substrates including cytosolic proteins of rat liver.

Protein Transport into Lysosomes

As the effect of ATP on the degradation of proteins by the intact lysosomes has been shown not to be caused

TABLE I.

Incorporation of ^{125}I-Proteins into Lysosomes

Incubation conditions	^{125}I-Proteins incorporated
	(cpm)
0°C	20
No additions, 37°C	1,220
ATP + Mg^{2+}(20 mM), 37°C	1,630

The incubation mixtures were the same as described in Fig. 3. After incubation for 30 min, the amount of ^{125}I-labeled cytosolic proteins incorporated into the lysosomes was determined as described in the text. The results are the averages of duplicate experiments, and zero-time control value (1,650 cpm) has been subtracted from all the values.

TABLE II.

Effect of ATP Plus Mg^{2+} on Acid Phosphatase

Concentrations of ATP and Mg^{2+}	Enzymatic Activity	
(mM)	Intact lysosomes	Triton-treated lysosomes
0	0.03	0.28
2.5	0.02	0.16
5	0.02	0.14
10	0.02	0.12
20	0.02	0.11

Acid phosphatase was assayed by the method of Andersch and Szcypinski (17) with p-nitrophenylphosphate as substrate at pH 4.8. Sucrose was added to make the final concentration of 0.25M in the reaction mixtures. Results are expressed as µmoles product formed/mg lysosomal protein/min.

by the direct activation of cathepsins within the lysosomes, the cause of the effect of ATP must be either
that ATP enhances penetration of substrate molecules
into lysosomes or that ATP facilitates release of
cathepsins into the reaction medium.

In an attempt to distinguish these alternatives,
we investigated the effect of ATP on the release of
proteases from intact lysosomes. Preincubation of
intact lysosomes in the presence or absence of ATP
plus Mg^{2+} did not cause any significant change in the
amount of proteolytic enzymes released into the medium
(Fig. 4). Thus ATP does not stimulate the release of
lysosomal cathepsins into the reaction medium.

The direct demonstration that ATP stimulates the
penetration of substrate proteins into lysosomes was
achieved by the use of ^{125}I-labeled liver cytosolic
proteins. The ^{125}I-labeled proteins were incubated
with intact lysosomes in an isotonic sucrose medium
in the presence or absence of ATP plus Mg^{2+}. The
incubation was stopped by chilling the reaction mixture in an ice bath, and the lysosomes were recovered
by centrifuging at 15,000 x g for 10 min. The sedi-
mented lysosomes were gently homogenized with an isotonic sucrose in phosphate buffer (0.05 M, pH 7.0)
and centrifugation was repeated. The efficiency of
removal of ^{125}I-radioactivity adsorbed on the surface
of the lysosomal membranes by repeated washings was
determined by measuring the radioactivity of the
supernatant after each centrifugation. Three washings
were found to be sufficient to remove most non-speci-
fically adsorbed radioactivities. Thus, the radioactivities incorporated into the lysosomes were counted
after three such washings and the results are presented
in Table I. Practically no radioactivity was incorporated on incubation at 0°C. On incubation at 37°C,
a considerable amount of radioactivity was incorporated
into the lysosomes and this was significantly stimulated by the addition of ATP plus Mg^{2+}. The degree
of stimulation in this experiment may seem to be less
pronounced than one would expect from the marked effect of ATP on the proteolysis (Fig. 3). One explanation for this is that the final radioactivity retained

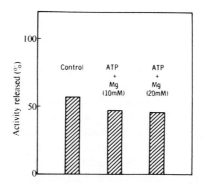

Figure 4: Effect of preincubation on the release of the proteolytic activity from lysosomes in the presence or absence of ATP plus Mg^{2+}. The intact lysosomes were preincubated in 0.25M sucrose, 0.05M acetate buffer (pH 4.5) at 37°C for 30 min. After the preincubation, the suspension was centrifuged at 15,000 x g for 20 min, and the catheptic activities were assayed for both the supernatant and the precipitate. The fraction of the activity in the supernatant over the combined activity of the supernatant and precipitate is regarded as the released activity during the preincubation.

TABLE III.

Effect of ATP Plus Mg^{2+} on β-Glucuronidase

Concentrations of ATP and Mg^{2+}	Enzymatic Activity	
(mM)	Intact lysosomes	Triton-treated lysosomes
0	0.76	9.7
2.5	0.76	–
5	0.76	–
10	0.76	9.9
20	0.76	–

β-Glucuronidase was assayed by the method of Gianetto and deDuve (18) with phenolphthalein glucuronide as substrate at pH 5.2. Sucrose (0.25M) was added to all the reaction mixtures. Results are expressed as μmoles product formed/mg lysosomal protein/min.

in the lysosomes does not represent the total amount
of the incorporated proteins, as the intralysosomal
proteolysis has been proceeding until the termination
of the incubation, and the repeated washings afterward
would have removed the degradation products from the
lysosomes. We may conclude from the data shown in
Table I that proteins are transported into the lysosomes by a temperature- and ATP-dependent process.

Effect on Other Lysosomal Enzymes

The experiments described above have established
that ATP affects lysosomal proteases by changing the
penetration of substrate proteins into lysosomes. Does
this phenomenon occur in the case of other lysosomal
enzymes?

The effect of ATP and Mg^{2+} on lysosomal acid phosphatase was studied. As is shown in Table II, the
addition of ATP and Mg^{2+} in equimolar concentrations
had no effect upon acid phosphatase activities in intact lysosomes, whereas in 'Triton'-treated lysosomes,
increasing concentrations of ATP and Mg^{2+} caused progressive inhibition of the enzymatic activities. This
inhibition should be caused by ATP which by itself
serves as a substrate for phosphatase and acts as a
competitive inhibitor against p-nitrophenylphosphate.
The observation that ATP and Mg^{2+} had no effect in the
intact lysosomes indicates that the penetration of p-
nitrophenylphosphate into lysosomes is unaffected by
ATP.

The effect of ATP and Mg^{2+} on another lysosomal
enzyme, β-glucuronidase, was also studied. The results
given in Table III show that ATP plus Mg^{2+} causes
no change in β-glucuronidase activity in the intact
lysosomes. The addition of 'Triton' to the system
caused elevation of enzymatic activity because membranous structures were disrupted, but ATP had no
effect upon the activity. Thus, unlike proteins, the
penetration of small molecular substrates, phenolphthalein glucuronide in the case of β-glucuronidase
and p-nitrophenylphosphate in the case of acid phosphatase, does not seem to be affected by ATP. This

result indicates that the action of ATP is specific
to macromolecules. We have obtained supporting evidence that the activity of acid ribonuclease, another
lysosomal enzyme acting on macromolecular RNA, is
stimulated by ATP (result not shown here).

All these features of the ATP effects point to a
similarity between the behavior of the intact lysosomes and the phenomenon of pinocytosis. We can envisage that protein and other macromolecules of the
cytoplasm are translocated into the lysosomes by the
process of "pinocytosis" and that those macromolecules
are degraded inside the lysosomes. The energy requirement for this process is readily understandable. The
possible involvement of a lysosomal membrane-bound
adenosine triphosphatase in controlling the release
of certain lysosomal enzymes has been suggested (12).

Physiological Significance

Finally, a question may be raised as to the physiological role of lysosomes in the intracellular protein
degradation in vivo. Lysosomal cathepsins are now
believed to make the greatest contribution to the overall process of intracellular protein degradation.
Haider & Segal (13), in studying the inactivating system of alanine aminotransferase and arginase in rat
liver, have provided evidence that the lysosomal preparation is responsible for the turnover of these enzymes in vivo. Auricchio & Liguori (14) studied the
inactivation of tyrosine aminotransferase in rat liver
homogenate and reached a similar conclusion. A relatively low pH optimum for the action of cathepsins
found in vitro may seem unphysiological for the activity in vivo, but the local hydrogen ion concentrations of the intralysosomal milieu within the living
cells could be similar to the situation in vitro. If
our finding that ATP promotes the transport of liver
cytosolic proteins into the lysosomes (Table I) holds
true in the situation in vivo, then the ATP concentration in the cytosol would influence the rate of intracellular protein degradation and thus the apparent
energy requirement for the protein degradation described
earlier in this article may be explained.

246

The physiological concentration of ATP in rat liver tissue has been reported to be in the range of 1 to 2 μmoles per g of the tissue (15). Our study has shown that the addition of ATP plus Mg^{2+} to intact lysosomes causes an almost linear increase in proteolytic activity up to 10 mM. The normal range of hepatic ATP concentrations, therefore, lies within the linear portion of the stimulatory effect and any changes in ATP concentrations would result in a change in the rate of protein degradation in vivo.

Data contained in this article were taken from M. Hayashi et al., Nature New Biology 242, 163 (1973).

References

1. Simpson, M. V.   J. Biol. Chem. 201, 143 (1953).
2. Steinberg, D. & Vaughan, M.   Arch. Biochem. Biophys. 65, 93 (1956).
3. Korner, A. & Tarver, H.   J. Gen. Physiol. 41, 219 (1957).
4. Penn, N. W.   Biochim. Biophys. Acta 37, 55 (1960).
5. Umaña, C. R.   Proc. Soc. Exptl. Biol. Med. 135, 925 (1970).
6. Brostrom, C. O. & Jeffay, H.   J. Biol. Chem. 245, 4001 (1970).
7. Huisman, W., Bouma, J. M. B., & Gruber, M. Biochim. Biophys. Acta 297, 93 (1973).
8. Goldspink, D. F. & Goldberg, A. L.   Biochem. J. 134, 829 (1973).
9. Hunter, J. E. & Harper, A. E.   Proc. Soc. Exptl. Biol. Med. 144, 731 (1973).
10. Coffey, J. W. & deDuve, C.   J. Biol. Chem. 243, 3255 (1968).
11. Sawant, P. L., Desai, I. D. & Tappel, A. L. Biochim. Biophys. Acta 85, 93 (1964).
12. Malbica, J. O.   Proc. Soc. Exptl. Biol. Med. 137, 1140 (1971).
13. Haider, M. & Segal, H. L.   Arch. Biochem. Biophys. 148, 228 (1972).
14. Auricchio, E. & Liguori.   FEBS Letters 12, 329 (1971).

15. Shull, K. H., McConomy, J., Vogt, M., Castillo,
    A. & Farber, E.   J. Biol. Chem. 241, 5060
    (1966).
16. Greenwood, F. C. & Hunter, W. M.   Biochem. J. 89,
    114 (1963).
17. Andersch, M. A. & Szcypinski, A. J.   Amer. J.
    Clin. Pathol. 17, 571 (1947).
18. Gianetto, R. & deDuve, C.   Biochem. J. 59, 433
    (1955).

The Inhibition of Cellular Protein Degradation in Rat Fibroblasts

Brian Poole

The Rockefeller University
New York, New York 10021

This paper will describe the results of some experiments on the degradation of cellular protein in confluent monolayers of rat fibroblasts. Proteins with slow and those with rapid turnover rates were labeled selectively with different isotopic forms of leucine in the same cell by a modification of the technique of Arias et al. (2). When fibroblasts are exposed to medium containing labeled leucine for an extended period, the labeled leucine becomes incorporated into all cellular proteins. When the cells are then washed and placed in unlabeled medium, those proteins with rapid rates of turnover are broken down and resynthesized from unlabeled leucine, leaving the labeled leucine in those proteins with slow rates of turnover. When the cells are then exposed for a short period to medium containing leucine labeled with another isotope, this isotope becomes incorporated chiefly into those proteins with rapid rates of turnover. The results of such a procedure are illustrated in Fig. 1. At the end of the short labeling period, the cells were washed and placed in unlabeled medium. The rate of release of the two isotopes into the medium in trichloroacetic acid (TCA) soluble form was then measured. At the end of the experiment the washed cells were dissolved in basic deoxycholate solution. In this Figure, and in all subsequent similar Figures, the label TCA-soluble in the medium is expressed as a fraction of the total label recovered in the medium and in the cells.

In the right-hand graph of Fig. 1, we see the output into the medium of label incorporated during the long labeling period (label derived from the breakdown of proteins with slow rates of turnover). The rate of output of this label was about 2% per hour and the rate did not change appreciably during the two-hour period of the experiment. There were no significant amounts of this label TCA-insoluble in the medium or TCA-soluble in the cells.

In the left-hand graph of Fig. 1, we see the output into the medium of TCA-soluble label incorporated during the short labeling period (derived from the breakdown of proteins with rapid rates of turnover) and the changes that occurred in the quantity of this label TCA-soluble in the cells. At zero time almost 15% of the total label in the system was in the cells in TCA-soluble form. However, during the first few minutes of the experiment, the amount of TCA-soluble label in the cells dropped rapidly. During this time the TCA-soluble label in the medium increased rapidly by about the amount lost by the cells. Then the TCA-soluble label in the medium continued to increase at a rapid rate until after 2 hours almost 30% of the total label in the system had been released into the medium. During this 2 hours the rate of release decreased progressively as the specific activity of the proteins with rapid rates of turnover decreased. Gel filtration of the TCA-soluble label in the medium indicated that the isotope was still chiefly in the form of leucine with a small fraction of degradation products but no higher molecular weight material. We have seen the apparent rapid loss from the cells into the medium of TCA-soluble label. The inhibition of protein synthesis did not affect the output of label nor did increasing the medium content in cold leucine. These observations suggest that leucine reutilization does not occur to any significant extent in this system and we can measure in the same cells the true rates of breakdown of proteins with rapid and those with slow rates of turnover.

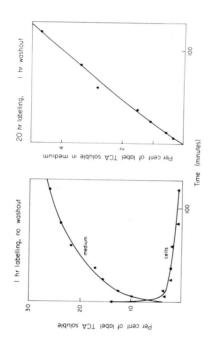

Fig. 1. Kinetics of degradation of cellular proteins. ●, TCA-soluble radioactivity in the medium (percent of total); ▲, TCA-soluble radioactivity in cells (percent of total).

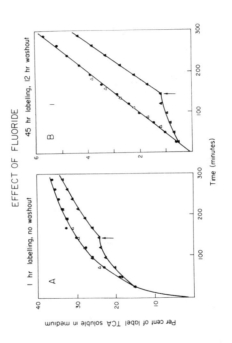

Fig. 2. Effect of 10 mM fluoride on cellular protein degradation. ●, control; ▲, fluoride. At the time indicated by the arrow, the medium was replaced by control medium.

The requirement of energy for cellular protein breakdown is well documented (7). Consequently, we studied the effect of a number of metabolic inhibitors on the rate of protein breakdown in fibroblasts. The most effective inhibitor at nontoxic concentration was found to be fluoride. Figure 2 shows the effect of this inhibitor on the degradation of cellular proteins of rapid turnover (left-hand graph) and slow turnover (right-hand graph). The degradation of both classes of protein was inhibited progressively until, after 150 minutes, degradation had almost ceased. At 150 minutes, when the cells were washed and placed in fresh medium without fluoride (arrow), protein degradation resumed with no indication of a lag period. To demonstrate the immediate reversal of fluoride inhibition, the experimental points after 150 minutes have been replotted (open symbols) with a time shift.

In order to determine whether the inhibitory effect of fluoride on cellular protein degradation was an inhibition of glycolysis resulting in a depletion of the cellular energy supply, we measured the rates of protein degradation and ATP levels in double-labeled fibroblasts treated with fluoride and iodoacetate. The results of this experiment are plotted in Fig. 3. Fluoride at a concentration of 10 mM caused about a 50% decrease in cellular ATP and a substantial decrease in the amount of label released from cellular proteins in 2 hours. Iodoacetate, on the other hand, caused a drastic decrease in cellular ATP and only a modest decrease in the rate of breakdown of cellular proteins. Consequently, the inhibitory effect of fluoride on protein degradation must involve some mechanism more specific than simply a reduction in the cellular energy supply. From the small effect of iodoacetate on the protein degradation while ATP levels were severely reduced, we can conclude that the process of cellular protein degradation requires rather low levels of ATP. It is noteworthy that the small effect of iodoacetate of protein degradation applied both to the proteins of slow and to

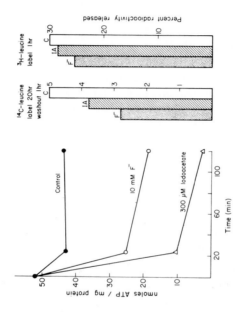

Fig. 3. Parallel measurements of ATP and cellular protein degradation. Bars indicate radioactivity in medium after 2 hr (percent of total). C, control; IA, iodoacetate; F, fluoride.

those of rapid turnover. If the inhibitory effect of iodoacetate is the consequence of its effect on energy metabolism, then energy must be required for the degradation of both classes of protein.

Chloroquine has been reported, on the basis of fluorescent microscopy, to be concentrated within lysosomes (1). It appears to inhibit hemoglobin digestion within the secondary lysosomes of plasmodia (5), and this may account for its antimalarial activity. Also it has been reported to stimulate autophagy in mammalian cells in culture (4). Consequently we examined the effect of this compound on cellular protein degradation in fibroblasts. The results of this experiment are shown in Fig. 4. There was a distinct inhibition of the degradation of proteins with rapid rates of turnover and of those with slow rates of turnover. When the cellular content of chloroquine was measured it was found that the concentration of this compound in the cells was several hundred times that in the medium. This means that under the conditions of Fig. 4, the average concentration of chloroquine in cell water was about 20 mM. If, as has been reported (1), the chloroquine was in the lysosomes, then the concentraion there must have been very much higher. In order to confirm the intracellular localization of chloroquine, we subjected chloroquine treated fibroblasts to subcellular fractionation by sucrose density gradient centrifugation. The results of this fractionation are shown in Fig. 5. The solid line shows the density distributions of marker enzymes from chloroquine treated cells, the dotted line those from the control cells. The density distributions of cytochrome oxidase (mitochondrial marker) and catalase were unaffected by the chloroquine treatment. There may have been a very slight shift of 5'-nucleotidase (plasma membrane marker) to higher density, but the most dramatic effect on the marker enzyme distributions was shown by the two lysosomal marker enzymes, acid phosphatase and N-acetyl-β-glucosaminidase. These two enzymes were shifted to lower densities by the chloroquine treatment. This is exactly what was

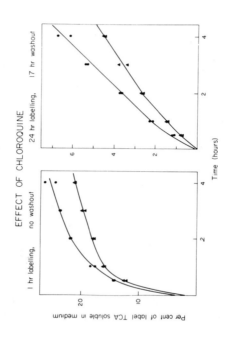

Fig. 4. The effect of 100 μM chloroquine on cellular protein degradation. ●, control; ▲, chloroquine.

256

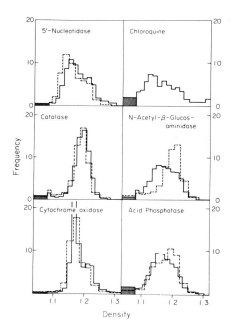

Figure 5: Isopycnic equilibration of fibroblast post-nuclear supernatant fraction in a zonal rotor (3). Solid lines, fibroblasts exposed to 100 μM chloroquine for 2 hr; dotted lines, control fibroblasts.

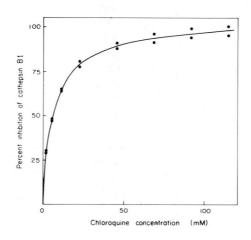

Fig. 6.   Inhibition of cathepsin B₁ by chloroquine.

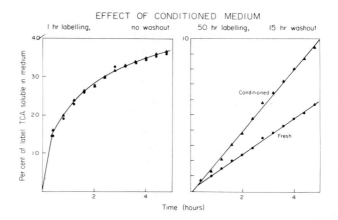

Fig. 7.   The effect of conditioned medium on cellular protein degradation.

to be expected if the lysosomes contain chloroquine.
In a sucrose gradient the lysosomal content and the
gradient solution are in osmotic equilibrium. Since
each chloroquine molecule carries with it two coun-
terions, lysosomes containing chloroquine would take
up water and become less dense. Most of the chloroquine entered the gradient and equilibrated at a
density slightly lower than that of the lysosomal
markers. This probably results from a variation in
the amount of chloroquine in individual lysosomes.
Those lysosomes with the most chloroquine would be
expected to have the lowest equilibrium densities.
Thus, the results of the subcellular fractionation
confirm the morphological results of Allison & Young
(1). The chloroquine within the fibroblasts appears
to be contained within lysosomes.

Even considering the dilatation of the vacuolar
system that results from chloroquine treatment, the
chloroquine concentration within the lysosomes must
have been on the order of 50 to 100 mM. We have
tested the effect of chloroquine on the activity of
a number of lysosomal cathepsins. The most dramatic
effects we found were on the activity of cathepsin B_1,
probably the most important lysosomal protease for
primary proteolytic attack on proteins. The concentration dependence of the inhibition of cathepsin B_1
by chloroquine is shown in Fig. 6. Half maximal inhibition occurred at about 5 mM and very little
activity remained at the concentration of chloroquine
we calculate to be within the lysosomes. Consequently
the most probable explanation of the effect of chloroquine on the degradation of cellular proteins is an
inhibition of proteolysis after the cellular protein
had entered lysosomes. If this explanation is true,
it means that proteins of both slow and rapid turnover
are degraded within lysosomes.

The inhibition of cellular protein degradation by
the three compounds described above, fluoride, iodoacetate and chloroquine, applied equally to the proteins of slow and to those of rapid turnover. This
suggests that there are common steps in the mechanism

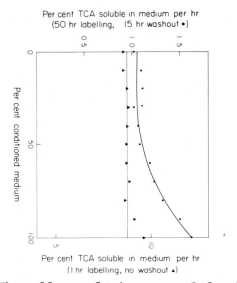

Figure 8: The effect of mixtures of fresh and
conditioned medium on protein degradation.

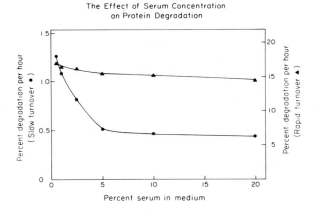

Fig. 9. The effect of serum on protein degradation.

TABLE I.

Medium	Percent Label Output in 2 Hours ± S.D.	
	Rapid Turnover	Slow Turnover
Control	20.9 ± .4	1.85 ± .17
– Amino Acids	20.4 ± .7	2.62 ± .36

260

of degradation of these two classes. However, there
are a number of treatments that have a differential
effect on the degradation of the two classes of protein. Figure 7 shows the difference in rates of cellular protein degradation when double-labeled fibroblasts were placed in fresh medium or in conditioned
medium (in which cells have been growing for several
days). Proteins with slow rates of turnover were
degraded about 50% more rapidly in the presence of
conditioned medium than they were in fresh medium,
while the rate of degradation of proteins with rapid
rates of turnover was identical in the two media.
Figure 8 shows the rate of degradation of the two
classes of protein in various mixtures of fresh and
conditioned medium. As would be expected from the
results of Fig. 7, the rate of degradation of proteins
with rapid rates of turnover was independent of medium
composition, while that of proteins with slow rates of
turnover was more rapid in the conditioned medium. It
is clear from Fig. 8 that the difference between the
two media resulted from inhibitory factors in the
fresh medium. The addition of small amounts of fresh
medium to pure conditioned medium resulted in a change
in the rate of degradation, while the addition of
small amounts of conditioned medium to fresh medium
had no effect.

Figure 9 shows the effect of serum concentration
on the degradation of the two classes of protein.
There was little or no effect on the degradation of
proteins with rapid rates of turnover, but there was
a dramatic inhibitory effect of serum on the degradation of proteins with slow rates of turnover.

Finally, Table I shows the effect of the medium
content in amino acids on the degradation of the two
classes of protein. Amino acids inhibited the degradation of proteins with slow rates of turnover but
had no effect on the degradation of proteins with
rapid rates of turnover. A similar effect has been
reported in the perfused rat liver (8).

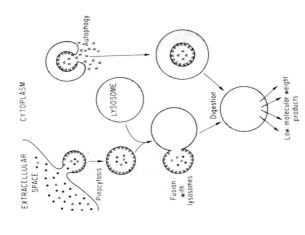

Fig. 10. Comparison of pinocytosis and hypothetical mechanism of cellular protein sequestration by lysosomes.

Three chemically very different substances, fluoride, iodoacetate, and chloroquine, inhibit the degradation of cellular proteins of slow and of fast turnover. This suggests very strongly that there are common steps in the mechanism of degradation of these two classes of protein by chloroquine, essentially all of which is inside lysosomes, suggests that at least some of both classes of protein are degraded within lysosomes. However, serum and amino acids inhibited the degradation of those proteins that turn over slowly without any effect on the degradation of those that turn over rapidly. It is known that some cellular proteins are degraded within lysosomes after autophagic vacuole formation. A portion of cytoplasm, often containing recognizable structures like mitochondria or rough endoplasmic reticulum, becomes surrounded by a membrane to form an autophagic vacuole. This vacuole then fuses with lysosomes and the contents of the vacuole are digested. It is not known what fraction of total cellular protein digestion occurs in this way. Autophagic vacuoles are seen more frequently in pathological situations but they do occur in apparently healthy cells. There is no evidence for specificity in autophagic vacuole formation. The portion of cytoplasm enclosed within the vacuoles seems no different from any other. Autophagic vacuole formation is somewhat analogous to phagocytosis where a small lump of material, such as a bacterium, is endocytized. Pinocytosis, the process by which soluble extracellular proteins are transported into the cell and then into lysosomes, is a highly specific process (6). Cells exposed to a mixture of proteins in the medium will endocytize and digest different proteins at very different rates, just as cells somehow digest their own constituent proteins at different rates. The selectivity in this process depends on specific receptors on the plasma membrane. This is illustrated on the left-hand side of Fig. 10, where the filled and open circles represent two different protein species in the medium. The protein represented by the open circles adsorbs on the

membrane and it is digested more rapidly than the
other protein. On the right-hand side of Fig. 10 is
illustrated an analogous process whereby cellular
proteins adsorb to varying degrees outside the lysosomal membrane and then are transferred into the
lysosomes by invaingation of the lysosomal membrane
followed by pinching off. In this mechanism the
selective binding sites are on what is topologically
the other side of the membrane. Small vesicles are
frequently found within lysosomes, but otherwise there
is no experimental evidence for this hypothetical
mechanism for the selective sequestration of cellular
proteins within lysosomes. However, the idea is very
attractive because of the formal analogy with the
well-studied process of pinocytosis and because it
explains the occurrence of different turnover rates
for different cellular proteins.

Supported by Grant HD-05065 from the U. S. Public
Health Service.

References

1. Allison, A. C. & Young, M. R.   Life Sciences 3,
      1407 (1964).
2. Arias, I. M., Doyle, D. & Schimke, R. T.   J.
      Biol. Chem. 244, 3303 (1969).
3. Beaufay, H.   La centrifugation en gradient de
      densite.   Ceuterick S. A., Louvain (1966).
4. Fedorko, M. E., Hirsch, J. G. & Cohn, Z. A.   J.
      Cell Biol. 38, 392 (1968).
5. Homewood, C. A., Warhurst, D. C., Peters, W. &
      Baggaley, V. C.   Nature 235, 50 (1972).
6. Jacques, P.   in Lysosomes in Biology and Pathology
      (J. T. Dingle & H. B. Fell, eds.).   North-
      Holland Publishing Co., Amsterdam.   Vol. 2,
      p. 395 (1969).
7. Poole, B.   in Enzyme Synthesis and Degradation in
      Mammalian Systems (M. Rechcigl, Jr., ed.)
      Karger, Basel, p. 375 (1971).
8. Woodside, K. H. & Mortimer, G. E.   J. Biol. Chem.
      247, 6474 (1972).

REGULATORY EFFECTS OF INSULIN, GLUCAGON AND AMINO ACIDS ON HEPATIC PROTEIN TURNOVER IN ASSOCIATION WITH ALTERATIONS OF THE LYSOSOMAL SYSTEM

Glenn E. Mortimore and Alice N. Neely

Department of Physiology
The Milton S. Hershey Medical Center
The Pennsylvania State University
Hershey, Pennsylvania 17033

The protein content of liver, as of any tissue, is determined by the balance between overall rates of protein synthesis and degradation. One may regard these general rates as reflecting simply the turnover of a great diversity of individual proteins, some of which are known to be controlled specifically. It is also true that the protein content varies widely under physiological conditions (1-3) and can be influenced directly by hormonal and nonhormonal agents (4-8). The magnitude and rapidity of these effects suggests that a comparatively large fraction of liver protein is regulated as a class on a moment-to-moment basis. Since free amino acid pools are strongly affected by this regulation and may in part determine it (7), it is probable that protein turnover plays a major role in maintaining the availability of amino acids for processes such as gluconeogenesis and obligatory routes of protein synthesis during periods of a variable supply of exogenous amino acids.

In this communication we shall review briefly our methods for the measurement of general protein synthesis and degradation in the isolated, perfused rat liver and describe effects of insulin, glucagon and amino acids on these parameters and on some associated lysosomal alterations.

Measurement of Protein Synthesis and Degradation in the Perfused Rat Liver. Valine has proved to be a useful marker for measuring protein turnover in the perfused rat liver. Except for its entry into and release from protein, valine is virtually inert metabolically (6,9). Thus net alterations of the total pool of free valine provide a means for monitoring moment-to-moment changes in the content of valine in peptide linkage. While these metabolic properties are shared by the other two branched-chain amino acids, leucine and isoleucine (9), valine has the additional advantage of being relatively easy to isolate and measure by paper chromatography (6).

A major difficulty that has been encountered in studies of the regulation of protein turnover has been to discriminate between effects of synthesis vis-a-vis degradation. Since the precursor pool for synthesis is under continuous dilution by endogenous proteolysis (10-14), its specific radioactivity after equilibration with label in the medium may be considerably lower than that of the extracellular pool. This difficulty is further complicated by a possible compartmentation of intracellular amino acids (Fig. 1). Studies of intracellular valine in the rat liver in vivo and after perfusion have indicated that the precursor or equilibrating pool may have a higher specific radioactivity at physiological concentrations than that of the total extractable intracellular valine pool (13,14). The perfusion data suggested the presence of a compartmented pool of low specific activity, derived from proteolysis, which did not mix with the precursor pool and whose size was independent of external valine concentration (13). Thus estimates of protein synthesis based strictly on the specific activity of the total extractable valine pool could be too high.

Our approach to the measurement of protein synthesis and degradation in the perfused rat liver has been to minimize or, hopefully, eliminate the effect of these errors by the addition of high concentrations of valine to the perfusing medium. Our rationale was based on the observation that as external valine is increased,

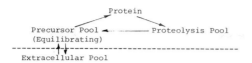

Figure 1. Hypothetical scheme showing major valine pools and pathways of valine flow in rat liver (13).

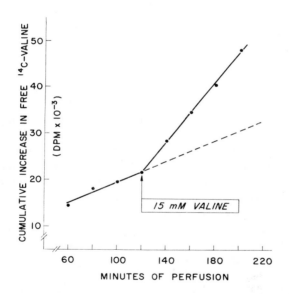

Figure 2: Effect of unlabeled 15 mM valine on the accumulation of (^{14}C)valine during perfusion of a rat liver previously labeled with L-(1-^{14}C) valine in vivo (13). The broken line depicts the linear course of accumulation in control perfusions, established previously (6,7).

267

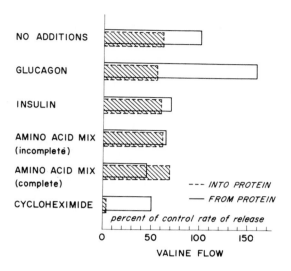

Figure 3: Effects of various agents on rates of incorporation of valine into and release from protein during rat liver perfusion. All rates are expressed as a percent of the mean rate of valine release in control perfused livers, which was estimated to be 0.3 μmole valine·min^{-1} per 100 g body weight, representing 3.8% per hr of the total pool of valine in peptide linkage (6,8). All effects are maximal and the data shown were obtained from the following sources: glucagon (8); insulin (6); incomplete amino acid mixture (7); complete amino acid mixture (7,8 and K. H. Woodside, personal communication); cycloheximide (K. H. Woodside, personal communication).

the equilibrating or precursor pool is increased proportionally (13). Thus errors introduced by compartmentation and the dilution of precursor amino acids by proteolysis are correspondingly reduced. Valine loading can be used either to inhibit competitively the reincorporation of labeled valine generated from the breakdown of protein in previously labeled livers, thus providing a measure of protein degradation, or to assess incorporation directly in pulse-label experiments where the valine load is labeled.

As illustrated by the broken line in Fig. 2, net rates of accumulation of [^{14}C]valine from previously labeled livers are constant after the first 60 min of perfusion. Since protein is the only source of label under these conditions, the specific radioactivity of the intracellular and extracellular valine pools will be equal (13). Furthermore, they have been shown to remain relatively constant after 60 min of perfusion (13). The unidirectional rate of valine release by proteolysis may thus be calculated from the accumulation of label in the presence of unlabeled 15 mM valine divided by the specific radioactivity of free valine prior to the addition of the valine load (13). The abrupt increase in the accumulation of label after the addition of valine in Fig. 2 represents label that would normally have been incorporated into protein. This increase, or the difference between the rates of accumulation prior to and after the addition of valine, may be used to calculate overall valine incorporation when divided by the specific radioactivity of free valine as in the above procedure. Previous studies have shown close agreement between rates of valine incorporation calculated in this manner and rates estimated directly in incorporation experiments from a labeled 15 mM valine pool (13). These rates (see Fig. 3) are in accord with estimates based on early rates of incorporation of [^{14}C]CO$_2$ into the guanidyl carbon of arginine in rats in vivo (11).

It is possible that the high concentration of valine used in these methods might have reduced protein synthesis as, for example, by interfering competitively

with the transport of certain key amino acids. Perfusion experiments run in the presence of a 15 mM
valine load, however, revealed no alterations in the
net accumulation of leucine or isoleucine or of steady-
state intracellular concentrations of most other amino
acids (13). Glutamine and glutamate were slightly
reduced, but these reductions were probably unrelated
to protein turnover per se. Since the metabolic behavior of leucine and isoleucine in liver is similar to
valine, any decrease in synthesis would have increased
their rates of accumulation unless protein degradation
were concurrently reduced by the same amount.

Effects of Insulin, Amino Acids and Glucagon on
General Protein Turnover. Our interest in the regulation of general protein turnover was generated from
early reports that insulin is capable of stimulating
the incorporation of labeled amino acids into liver
protein in vitro (15,16) and thus may serve as a regulator of general protein synthesis in this tissue.
Subsequent investigation using perfused rat livers
showed that the apparent stimulus to incorporation by
insulin was the consequence of an inhibitory action
on protein degradation which decreased the dilution
of the precursor amino acid pool, thereby increasing
the incorporation of label (6). As shown in Fig. 3
valine incorporation is not increased by insulin when
the effect of precursor pool dilution is minimized by
the addition of 15 mM valine.

The infusion of an incomplete mixture of amino acids,
patterned after the composition of an ovalbumin hydro-
lysate except for omission of valine, leucine, isoleucine, and tyrosine (7), mimicked the effect of insulin
by suppressing proteolysis without influencing valine
incorporation (Fig. 3). Additions of complete amino
acid mixtures, simulating the amino acid composition
of rat plasma at 10X normal concentrations, did stimulate incorporation to a small (12%) but significant
degree (7,8) and produced the greatest inhibition (55%)
of general protein degradation that we have yet observed
(K. H. Woodside, personal communication). Of further
interest is the fact that the addition of cycloheximide

$(1.8 \times 10^{-5}M)$, which inhibited valine incorporation by 93%, reduced proteolysis by 50% (K. H. Woodside, personal communication). Similar effects on protein degradation of inhibitors of synthesis have been reported (17-19) and are possibly mediated by increases in intracellular amino acids.

Glucagon is known to evoke a wide variety of responses in liver and among these is a strong catabolic effect on protein metabolism (4,5). Effects of this hormone that we have observed in liver perfusion studies are depicted in Fig. 3. Proteolysis was stimulated nearly 60%; valine incorporation was inhibited by 15% and net protein degradation, denoted by the blank area of the bars in Fig. 3, was more than doubled (8). In other experiments, not shown here, the inhibition of protein synthesis by glucagon was increased from 15 to nearly 40% in the presence of a complete mixture of amino acids (8), a finding which suggests that glucagon may play a dual role in the regulation of protein turnover under physiological circumstances.

A second set of conditions in which the rate of protein degradation is regularly increased is perfusion itself. In an earlier study we reported that proteolysis spontaneously increased rather abruptly after 20 to 30 min of perfusion and then remained elevated up to 180 min (6). This spontaneous increase which occurs in the absence of an elevation in the tissue level of cyclic AMP (20), is abolished by insulin (6) or the addition of amino acids (7). It is therefore reasonable to suppose that insulin and amino acids both serve in some way (or ways) to restrain general proteolysis in vivo. When this restraint is reduced by perfusion, degradation increases.

Lysosomal alterations. In seeking a mechanism which might explain these regulatory effects on proteolysis, we undertook a series of experiments based on findings of Deter and de Duve (21). Glucagon is a known inducer of autophagic vacuoles in rat liver (21,22), and an increase in the population of these lysosomal particles was shown by Deter and de Duve to enhance the sensitivity of lysosomes to osmotic and mechanical shock as

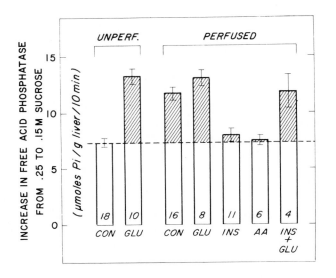

Figure 4: Alterations in the sensitivity of hepatic lysosomes to osmotic shock under various conditions (23). Osmotic sensitivity was assessed from the increase in free acid phosphatase obtained after reducing the concentration of sucrose in liver homogenates from 0.225 to 0.15M (23). Note error in labeling of the vertical coordinate. Values are means ± one S.E.; shaded areas depict increases above unperfused control values; the number of experiments for each group is given at the bottom of each bar. Abbreviations are: CON, control; GLU, glucagon; INS, insulin; AA, incomplete amino acid mixture.

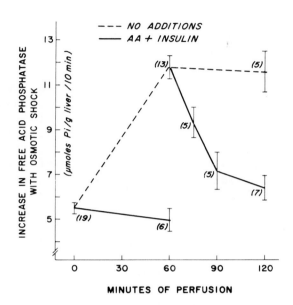

Figure 5: Reversal by an incomplete mixture of amino
    acids + insulin of the spontaneous increase in
    osmotic sensitivity during rat liver perfusion
    (23). Release of acid phosphatase following
    osmotic shock was assessed as in Fig. 4. Separate
    perfusions were run for each time-point and the
    numbers of experiments are given in parentheses;
    the plotted values are means ± one S.E.

manifested by a decrease in the latency of lysosomal enzymes. Presumably the effect was related to the larger size of autophagic vacuoles in comparison with normal dense bodies, which rendered the former more susceptible to osmotic and mechanical stress (21).

It can be seen in Fig. 4 that the administration of glucagon to rats in vivo increased appreciably the amount of free acid phosphatase measured in liver homogenates after osmotic shock. The latter was determined from the increase in free enzyme activity which occurred after reducing the sucrose concentration from 0.225 to 0.15M (23). Of particular interest to us was the fact that perfusion alone acted like glucagon to enhance osmotic sensitivity. Additions of insulin or incomplete mixtures of amino acids strongly inhibited the effect of perfusion. While glucagon alone failed to elicit a significant response in perfused livers, an effect was observed in the presence of insulin. In experiments reported elsewhere cycloheximide at a concentration of 1.8×10^{-5}M inhibited completely the spontaneous increase in osmotic sensitivity with perfusion (23). Effects of glucagon on osmotic sensitivity (23) and on proteolysis (8) were not blocked under these conditions.

It should be emphasized that no alterations in total acid phosphatase were noted in these studies nor did perfusion itself or the administration of glucagon increase free acid phosphatase in the initial isotonic homogenates as has been reported elsewhere (21,24,25). We may conclude from the latter findings that the integrity of the lysosomal membrane in the intact cell was not compromised either by perfusion or the addition of glucagon during perfusion.

The time-course of osmotic sensitivity during control perfusion is depicted by the broken line shown in Fig. 5. The increase in osmotic sensitivity reached a maximum by 60 min and then remained constant through 120 min of perfusion. Additions of insulin and amino acids at the start prevented the increase in sensitivity and when added at 60 min, sharply reversed it. In other experiments the removal of insulin and amino

TABLE I.

Cumulative Distribution of β-Acetylglucosaminidase

as Percent of Total

Fractions	Unperfused(6)	Perfused, No Additions(6)	Perfused, Amino Acids + Insulin(6)
1-5	5.9 ± 1.2	18.4 ± 2.1	6.6 ± 3.3
1-10	36.3 ± 2.3	56.0 ± 1.2	38.6 ± 3.3
1-15	80.0 ± 1.4	88.2 ± 1.0	83.1 ± 1.4
1-20	93.5 ± 0.7	95.1 ± 0.8	93.9 ± 1.0
1-25	100	100	100

Effect of liver perfusion with and without additions of an incomplete amino acid mixture + insulin on the distribution of β-acetylglucosaminidase after equilibrium density centrifugation in linear sucrose gradients (26). Mitochondrial + lysosome subcellular fractions were layered on linear 35-70% sucrose gradients. The particles were spun to equilibrium in an SW-41 rotor (Beckman) at 15.4×10^6 g x min. Fractions were collected from the bottom of the tubes (fraction 1 = greatest density) and the enzyme was assayed essentially as described by Barrett (29). The values shown are means ± one S.E. and the number of experiments are in parenthesis.

acids by changing to fresh medium after 60 min resulted
in a prompt rise in osmotic sensitivity to perfused
control levels (23). A similar pattern of response
has been observed with the use of another lysosomal
marker enzyme, β-acetylglucosaminidase (23). It thus
seems clear that these lysosomal alterations are related in some fundamental way to the presence or absence of hormones and substrate. The possibility
that tissue damage was involved to a significant
degree appears to be excluded.

Additional studies utilizing equilibrium density
centrifugation have revealed significant shifts in
lysosomal density that occurred under conditions similar to those producing alterations of osmotic sensitivity (26). At equilibrium the distribution of β-
acetylglucosaminidase in a linear sucrose gradient
produced a well-defined peak which overlapped, but
was clearly distinguishable from a protein peak con-
stituting the bulk of mitochondria. Cathepsin D was
distributed in the same manner. In Table I we show
effects of perfusion, both with and without additions
of insulin and amino acids, on the cumulative distribution of β-acetylglucosaminidase after density gradient fractionation. In comparison with unperfused
controls, perfusion per se caused a highly significant
shift in the distribution of the enzyme into the den-
ser gradient fractions ($p < .001$), an effect which
was completely eliminated by the administration of
insulin and the incomplete mixture of amino acids. No
shifts in the protein peak were observed and, as would
be expected, cathepsin D moved with β-acetylglucosaminidase.

Electron micrographic examination of perfused tissue has offered additional information as to the nature
of these lysosomal alterations (26). In control liver
perfused for 60 or 120 min in the absence of any additions to the medium, the number of lysosomal profiles
in the hepatocytes was increased 2-3 fold. The majority of these lysosomal elements, which were on the
average larger than dense bodies in unperfused liver,
contained an electron-dense core and a variable, but

well demarcated electron-lucent area. Perhaps the most significant finding was the lack of any conspicuous increase in true autophagic vacuoles, as shown by the lack of well-defined membrane inclusions. Typical autophagic vacuoles were observed, however, in perfused liver after glucagon treatment. It should be pointed out that these so-called perfusion elements could not be distinguished from normal lysosomal components in unperfused liver except for their greater abundance. Since these alterations were not observed in Kupffer cells, it is unlikely that they came about as a consequence of the endocytic phagocytic uptake of protein from the medium; rather their formation is more in keeping with some process involving the sequestration of intracellular material.

While the association between the regulatory effects on proteolysis and physical alterations of lysosomes supports the notion that the uptake of endogenous protein by the lysosomal system is directly involved in the mechanism of protein degradation, more information must be obtained before a link between these two sets of events can be established. Assuming that the final step in general proteolysis is the digestion of substrate protein by lysosomal proteases, products of digestion should accumulate in homogenates containing intact lysosomes as long as substrate is available and other requirements such as pH are met. Mego, for example, has demonstrated that the digestion of denatured albumin, taken up phagocytically by mouse liver, continues within lysosomes after cell disruption (27). We have shown that rates of leucine release in 0.225 M sucrose homogenates of perfused rat liver incubated at 37° correlates surprisingly well in a relative way with rates of proteolysis obtained during perfusion (28). Lysosomal fractions separated by equilibrium density centrifugation from previously labeled perfused livers have been shown to contain trichloracetic acid soluble radioactivity that was probably generated intralysosomally (26). Whether the leucine released in the above studies was also derived from the lysosome has not been established but it is reasonable to assume that it was. We do not know yet how well rates of proteolysis in homogenates will be able to account for rates measured in the intact liver. Such an accounting can only be made after we understand more fully the characteristics of lysosomal proteolysis.

References

1. Addis, T., Poo, L. J. & Lew, W. J. Biol. Chem. 115: 111 (1936).
2. Addis, T., Poo, L. J. & Lew, W. J. Biol. Chem. 115: 116 (1936).
3. Soberon, G. & Sanchez, Q. J. Biol. Chem. 236: 1602 (1961).
4. Izzo, J. L. & Glasser, S. R. Endocrinol. 68: 189 (1961).
5. Miller, L. L. Fed. Proc. 24: 737 (1965).
6. Mortimore, G. E. & Mondon, C. E. J. Biol. Chem. 245: 2375 (1970).
7. Woodside, K. H. & Mortimore, G. E. J. Biol. Chem. 247: 6474 (1972).
8. Woodside, K. H., Ward, W. F. & Mortimore, G. E. J. Biol. Chem. in press.
9. Miller, L. L. in Amino Acid Pools, J. T. Holten, ed., American Elsevier Publishing Co., New York, p. 708 (1962).
10. Loftfield, R. & Harris, A. J. Biol. Chem. 219: 151 (1956).
11. Swick, R. W. J. Biol. Chem. 231:751 (1958).
12. Gan, J. C. & Jeffay, H. Biochim. Biophys. Acta 148: 448 (1967).
13. Mortimore, G. E., Woodside, K. H. & Henry, J. E. J. Biol. Chem. 247: 2776 (1972).
14. Airhart, J., Vidrich, A. & Khairallah, E. A. Biochem. J., in press.
15. Penhos, J. C. & Krahl, M. E. Am. J. Physiol. 204: 140 (1963).
16. Mondon, C. E. & Mortimore, G. E. Am. J. Physiol. 212: 173 (1967).
17. Steinberg, D. & Vaughn, M. Biochim. Biophys. Acta 19: 584 (1956).

18. Hershko, A. & Tomkins, G. J. Biol. Chem. 246: 710 (1971).

19. Goldberg, A. Proc. Nat. Acad. Sci. U.S.A. 68: 362 (1971).

20. Exton, J. H., Robison, G. A., Sutherland, E. W. & Park, C. R. J. Biol. Chem. 246: 6166 (1971).

21. Deter, R. L. & deDuve, C. J. Cell Biol. 33: 437 (1967).

22. Ashford, T. P. & Porter, K. R. J. Cell Biol. 12: 198 (1962).

23. Neely, A. N., Nelson, P. B. & Mortimore, G. E. Biochim. Biophys. Acta 338: 458 (1974).

24. Guder, W., Frohlich, S., Patzelt, C. & Wieland, O. FEBS Letters 10: 215 (1970).

25. Vavrinkova, H. & Mosinger, B. Biochim. Biophys. Acta 231: 320 (1971).

26. Neely, A. N., Doctoral Dissertation (Physiol.), The Pennsylvania State University (1973).

27. Mego, J. L., Bertini, F. and McQueen, J. O. J. Cell Biol. 32: 699 (1967).

28. Mortimore, G. E., Neely, A. N., Cox, J. R. & Guinivan, R. A. Biochem. Biophys. Res. Commun. 54: 89 (1973).

29. Barrett, A. J. in "Lysosomes", J. T. Dingle (ed), American Elsevier Publishing Co., New York, p. 83 (1972).

This work was supported in part by Grant AM-16356 from the National Institute of Arthritis, Metabolism and Digestive Diseases.

CORRELATIONS BETWEEN IN VIVO TURNOVER AND IN VITRO INACTIVATION OF RAT LIVER ENZYMES

Judith S. Bond

Department of Biochemistry
Medical College of Virginia
Virginia Commonwealth University
Richmond, Virginia 23298

The factors or events that initiate the degradation
of specific intracellular proteins in vivo are not
understood. The initial phase in the degradation of
a protein might involve processes such as denaturation,
proteolysis, inactivation, any number of chemical
alterations of the protein molecule (e.g., deglycosyla-
tion, phosphorylation, acetylation) or a combination
of these processes. A study (1) of five soluble rat
liver enzymes indicated that enzymes with short half-
lives in vivo were more vulnerable to tryptic and
chymotryptic inactivation in vitro than enzymes with
comparatively long in vivo half-lives. The following
investigation was undertaken to extend those studies
to a larger group of enzymes with known in vivo half-
lives to compare: (a) the susceptibility of these
enzymes to inactivation by proteases, (b) their susceptibility to thermal inactivation in rat liver extracts and (c) their stability to acid environments
(incubation at pH 5). The aim of these studies was
to determine whether there are certain characteristics
which short-lived enzymes share to distinguish them
from long-lived enzymes.

Experimental Procedure

Male Holtzman rats (250–400 g) were killed by decapitation and livers perfused with NaCl (0.9%). Livers

were then homogenized at 4° with 0.15M KCl (1 g liver
+ 3 ml KCl) in a glass tube fitted with a Teflon Pestle
and centrifuged at 50,000 x g for 80 min. The resulting supernatant fraction was adjusted to pH 7 with
NaOH. These extracts were either used immediately or
stored at -20°.

Arginase activity was assayed by the method of Van
Slyke and Archibald (2). Lactate dehydrogenase was
assayed by the method described by Kornberg (3), glyceraldehyde-phosphate dehydrogenase as described by
Kuehl & Sumsion (4) and α-glycerophosphate dehydrogenase as described by Beisenherz et al. (5). Alanine
aminotransferase activity was determined by Assay
Method I described by Segal et al. (6) and tyrosine
aminotransferase according to Diamondstone (7). Glucokinase was assayed according to Salas et al. (8) and
catalase by Beers & Sizer's method (9). Serine dehydratase was assayed by the method of Pitot & Pries (10)
and dihydroorotase according to Bresnick et al. (11).
NAD$^+$ and NADH were determined by spectrophotometric
methods using yeast alcohol dehydrogenase (12). Protein was determined by the method of Lowry et al. (13)
with crystalline bovine albumin as a standard.

Trypsin (Type III: 2 x crystallized from bovine
pancreas), chymotrypsin (Type II: 3 x crystallized
bovine pancreas), subtilisin (Type VII: from <u>Bacillus</u>
<u>amylolique-faciens</u>) and pronase (Type VI: from <u>Strepto-</u>
<u>myces griseus</u>) were obtained from Sigma Chemical Co.,
St. Louis, Mo. Their proteolytic activity was assessed
by the method of Kunitz (14) using denatured casein,
or liver extracts as substrate; the increase in absor-
bance at 280 nm in trichloroacetic acid extracts or
ninhydrin-positive material (15) formed during incubation was measured.

Results

Inactivation by proteases. The enzymes that were
compared and their in vivo half-lives (t$_{1/2}$) as reported in the literature are listed in Table I. To
determine the effect of trypsin on inactivation of
these enzymes, rat liver extracts were incubated with

TABLE I. In vivo half-lives of rat liver enzymes (4,16,17)

Enzyme	Abbreviation	In vivo $t_{1/2}$ (days)
Lactate dehydrogenase (EC 1.1.1.27)	LDH	3.5, 16
Arginase (EC 3.5.3.1)	ARG	4 - 5
Glyceraldehyde-phosphate dehydrogenase (EC 1.2.1.12)	GPD	3.5
Alanine aminotransferase (EC 2.6.1.2)	AAT	3.0
α-Glycerophosphate dehydrogenase (EC 1.1.1.8)	αGD	4.0
Catalase (EC 1.11.1.6)	CAT	1.1, 2.2
Glucokinase (EC 2.7.1.2)	GK	0.5, 1.4
Dihydroorotase (EC 3.5.2.3)	DHO	0.5
Serine dehydratase (EC 4.2.1.13)	SD	0.12, 0.83
Tyrosine aminotransferase (EC 2.6.1.5)	TAT	0.08, 0.49

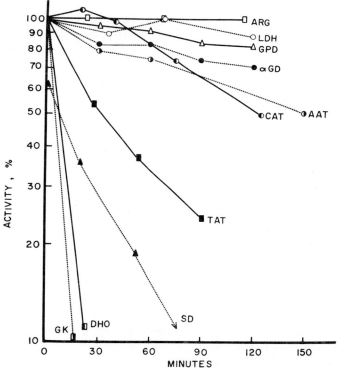

Figure 1: The effect of trypsin on enzyme activities in rat liver extracts. Extracts were incubated at 37° with trypsin (91 μg/ml) in 45 mM potassium phosphate buffer, pH 8. The incubation mixture had a final volume of 5.5 ml and contained 5.0 ml of extract to which 0.6 mM NAD^+ was added at the beginning of the incubation period and again after 40 min. The extract was adjusted to pH 8 before incubation with trypsin. Samples of the incubation mixture were removed at various times for enzyme assays. Activities are expressed as percent of initial activity in a buffered extract which did not contain trypsin. The enzymes assayed and abbreviations for the enzymes are as in Table I.

this protease and samples removed at various intervals for enzyme assays (Fig. 1). Arginase and lactate dehydrogenase were consistently found to be resistant to tryptic-inactivation under these conditions; glyceraldehyde-phosphate dehydrogenase and α-glycerophosphate dehydrogenase were stable as long as NAD$^+$ was present in incubation mixtures; whereas glucokinase and dihydroorotase were about 90% inactivated within 30 minutes of incubation. The other enzymes were inactivated to a moderate extent; the approximate order of inactivation (from least to most vulnerable) was as follows: alanine aminotransferase, catalase, tyrosine aminotransferase and serine dehydratase.

In control experiments, extracts were incubated in the absence of trypsin or in the presence of trypsin pre-mixed with trypsin inhibitor (in a ratio of 1:2). Under these conditions, at pH 8, all the enzymes were stable for at least two and one-half hours except for glyceraldehyde-phosphate dehydrogenase and glucokinase which were stable in some extracts but not in others. Glucose (100 mM) stabilized glucokinase, while ATP (6 mM), another substrate, had no effect. Glucokinase was rapidly inactivated by trypsin with or without glucose under the conditions shown in Fig. 1. Glyceraldehyde-phosphate dehydrogenase was stabilized by NAD$^+$ or NADH and was resistant to trypsin in the presence of both the reduced and oxidized form of the coenzyme. NAD$^+$, NADH and glucose did not affect the activities of any of the proteases used in these studies (measured by following the rate of digestion of casein).

Chymotrypsin, subtilisin and pronase were also used to assess the relative rates of inactivation of the enzymes (Table II). The enzymes are listed in order of decreasing half-life in vivo, as in Table I. The data indicate the following: (a) arginase and glyceraldehyde-phosphate dehydrogenase were resistant to all proteases; (b) alanine aminotransferase and α-glycerophosphate dehydrogenase were resistant to all except trypsin; (c) lactate dehydrogenase was stable to trypsin and chymotrypsin, but inactivated by subtilisin and pronase; (d) catalase and tyrosine aminotransferase were partially inactivated by all the proteases; (f) glucokinase, dihydroorotase and serine dehydratase were markedly inactivated by all proteases.

NAD$^+$ fully protected gluceraldehyde-phosphate dehydrogenase from inactivation by all of the proteases and partially protected α-glycerophosphate and lactate dehydrogenases. In other instances where ligands were tested for their ability to protect against trypsin; (a) alanine (30 mM), α-ketoglutaric acid (15 mM) and pyridoxal-5'-phosphate (0.1 mM) had no effect on the rate of inactivation of alanine aminotransferase; (b) tyrosine (3 mM) and α-ketoglutaric acid (10 mM) had no effect on the rate of tyrosine aminotransferase inactivation and (c) pyridoxal-5'-phosphate protected both tyrosine aminotransferase and serine dehydratase to a moderate extent (as reported previously (1)).

Inactivation by heat. For comparisons of the thermal stability of the enzymes, the rate of loss of enzyme activities in buffered extracts incubated at 45° was measured. Figure 2 shows the results from a single representative experiment. Arginase, alanine aminotransferase and α-glycerophosphate dehydrogenase were initially activated at 45°, to various extents in different extracts, and were then stable. Lactate dehydrogenase, glyceraldehyde-phosphate dehydrogenase and tyrosine aminotransferase were also stable, although the latter enzyme sometimes showed decreased activity directly after exposure to the 45° bath (not greater than 15% decrease). The other enzymes were unstable; glucokinase and dihydroorotase were most readily inactivated.

Dithioerythritol (2 mM) was included in several 45° incubation mixtures because a number of enzymes require sulfhydryl groups to remain reduced for activity. This reagent had no effect, however, on the stability of the enzymes. Dialysis of extracts for 40 hours against 0.15M KCl containing dithioerythritol (1 mM) and phosphate buffer (1 mM) also had no effect on the order of thermal stability of the enzymes.

In other experiments, pyridoxal-5'-phosphate (40 μM) did not stabilize serine dehydratase and glucose did

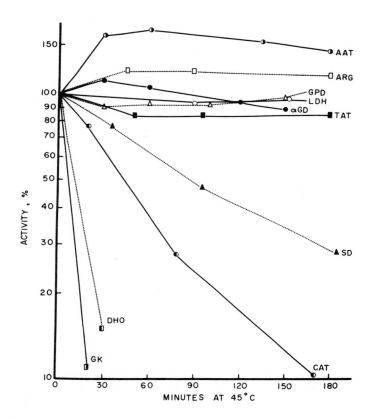

Figure 2: Thermal stability of enzymes in rat liver
extracts were incubated at 45° in 20 mM potassium
phosphate buffer, pH 7.3, with 0.6 mM NAD⁺. Portions of the incubation mixture were removed at
various times for enzyme assays. Activities are
expressed as percent of the activity in the buffered liver extract just prior to incubation at
45°. The enzymes assayed and abbreviations for
the enzymes are as in Table I.

not protect glucokinase. Carbamyl-aspartic (20 mM) partially protected dihydroorotase; the enzyme lost 70% activity in 90 min in the presence of carbamyl-aspartic acid.

Inactivation by acid. The stability of the enzymes at pH 5 was also compared (Fig. 3). The enzymes seemed to fall into two groups: those that were stable at pH 5, alanine aminotransferase, lactic dehydrogenase, glyceraldehyde-phosphate dehydrogenase, tyrosine aminotransferase and catalase; and those that were inactivated, glucokinase, dihydroorotase, serine dehydratase and arginase. α-Glycerophosphate dehydrogenase does not appear on Fig. 3 because there was no consistent pattern of inactivation at pH 5 in different extracts for this enzyme. In some instances it was completely stable for 2 hours, in others it was 80-90% inactivated within 30 min. The addition of NAD^+ to extracts did not affect the stability of the enzyme at pH 5. In other experiments where ligands were added to extracts, glucose (100 mM) did not protect glucokinase from inactivation at pH 5 and pyridoxal-5'-phosphate (40 μM) did not protect serine dehydratase at this pH.

DISCUSSION

Ligands affect the rates of inactivation of several enzymes in this study. The effects of NAD^+ on the stability of glyceraldehyde-phosphate dehydrogenase and α-glycerophosphate dehydrogenase are most marked. The concentrations of NAD^+ added to extracts were in the physiological range (18) and thus extracts with added NAD^+ simulate intracellular conditions better than those with no NAD^+ additions. For the other enzymes tested, ligands afford little or not protection.

There appears to be a general correlation between the resistance of enzymes to inactivation by proteases and heat and their stability in vivo. The long-lived enzymes (lactic dehydrogenase, arginase, glyceraldehyde-phosphate dehydrogenase, alanine aminotransferase and α-glycerophosphate dehydrogenase) are generally resistant

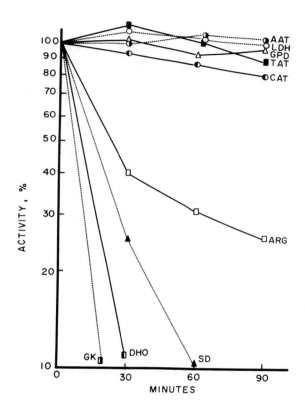

Figure 3: Enzyme stabilities at pH 5. Extracts were incubated at 37° with acetic acid buffer (50 mM, pH 5.0). The protein concentration in the incubation mixture was 8 mg per ml. Samples were removed with time and assayed for enzyme activity. The enzymes and abbreviations are the same as in Table I.

to proteases and heat while the short-lived enzymes
are generally inactivated partially or completely by
the proteases and heat, with the exception of tyrosine
aminotransferase. Johnson & Kenney (19) have noted
that the turnover of this enzyme is unusual in several
respects and it has been suggested that a specific and
labile "degrading enzyme" is involved in this instance.

There is evidence in the literature which indicates
that thermal instability is not an important factor in
initiating the degradation of intracellular proteins.
For instance, Kuehl & Sumsion (4) have found that the
rates of degradation of three glycolytic enzymes in
vivo are similar, while their thermal stabilities in
vitro are quite different. Also, Segal et al. (20),
studying alanine aminotransferase in rat tissues, have
concluded that degradation of this enzyme in vivo does
not depend on prior thermal denaturation. On the other
hand, Li & Knox (21) have concluded from studies on
tryptophan oxygenase from rat liver, that the initial
step in the degradation of this enzyme is akin to denaturation. It is possible that thermal instability
plays a role in determining in vivo instability for
short-lived enzymes but not for the long-lived enzymes
(e.g., the glycolytic enzymes and alanine aminotransferase).

No correlations between in vivo stability and stability in an acid environment (pH 5) have been found.
With respect to this parameter, three long-lived enzymes and two short-lived enzymes (tyrosine aminotransferase and catalase) are stable; three short-lived
enzymes and one long-lived enzyme (arginase) are unstable. No ligand protection could be demonstrated in
the instances where it has been tested. The stability
of the enzymes at low pH might have some importance
physiologically if lysosomes are involved in the initial stages of intracellular protein degradation. If
lysosomes act as sieves for intracellular contents as
has been suggested (22), the initiating event for
degradation may be stability in acid in lysosomes. The
results in this study indicate that this is not the
case. Preliminary studies on the effects of cathepsins

TABLE II. Effects of trypsin, chymotrypsin, subtilisin and pronase on the inactivation of enzymes in rat liver extracts.

Enzyme	Percentage of activity remaining after 90 min of incubation with:			
	trypsin	chymotrypsin	subtilisin	pronase
LDH	97	100	10	5
ARG	108	100	120	115
GPD	100	100	95	98
AAT	68	96	100	100
αGD	75	92	90	103
CAT	67	80	30	40
GK	0	0	0	0
DHO	0	10	20	10
SD	10	20	0	0
TAT	25	40	50	60

Extracts were incubated at 37° with one of the proteases (91 µg/ml) in 45 mM potassium phosphate buffer, pH 8, 0.6 mM NAD^+ and 100 mM glucose. Samples were removed before incubation and after 90 min for enzyme assays.

TABLE III. Molecular weights of rat liver enzymes and subunits (24,25,26)

Enzyme	In vivo $t_{1/2}$ (hours)	Molecular weight of:	
		enzyme	subunits
LDH	84-384	140,000	35,000
ARG	108	138,000	34,500
GPD	84	140,000	35,000
AAT	72	114,000	57,000
αGD	96	78,000	39,000
CAT	29	250,000	62,500
GK	24	50,000	----
DHO	12	----	----
SD	12	68,000	34,000
TAT	2	110,000	55,000

290

at pH 5 also indicate that those enzymes that are stable at pH 5 are also resistant to inactivation by cathepsins at this pH.

A general correlation between relative degradation rates and molecular size has been found by Dice et al. (23); larger proteins being degraded in vivo more rapidly than smaller ones. The larger proteins are also more susceptible to proteolysis with trypsin and pronase. These authors emphasize that the general trend may or may not be evident when a few specific enzymes are examined. For the enzymes used in the present study, the in vivo half-lives and the rates of inactivation by proteases do not correlate with the molecular weights or subunit weights (Table III).

It appears now that there are a number of factors which share in determining in vivo half-lives. The studies reported here confirm initial observations indicating that there is a trend for long-lived enzymes to be more resistant to inactivation by proteases than the short-lived enzymes. In addition, there is a general correlation between thermal stability of enzymes in extracts and in vivo stability. These studies are also consistent with the proposition that specific degradative enzymes are present for specific enzymes (such as tyrosine aminotransferase). These data indicate that all of these factors (proteases, thermal stability, coenzymes and specific degrading enzymes) are operative in the initiation of intracellular protein degradation and that the half-life of a protein molecule in vivo is at least in part determined by its physical and chemical properties.

ACKNOWLEDGEMENT

I thank Mrs. Kathleen McKay for excellent technical assistance. This work was supported by Grant GB31178 from the National Science Foundation.

References

1. Bond, J. S. Biochem. Biophys. Res. Commun. 43, 333 (1971).
2. Van Slyke, D. D. & Archibald, R. M. J. Biol. Chem. 165, 293 (1946).
3. Kornberg, A. in Methods in Enzymology (S. P. Colowick & N. O. Kaplan, eds.) Vol. I, 441 (1955).
4. Kuehl, L. & Sumsion, E. N. J. Biol. Chem. 245, 6616 (1970).
5. Beisenherz, G., Bucher, T. & Garbade, K. H. in Methods in Enzymology (S. P. Colowick & N. O. Kaplan, eds.) Vol. I, 391 (1955).
6. Segal, H. L., Beattie, D. S. & Hopper, S. J. Biol. Chem. 237, 1914 (1962).
7. Diamondstone, T. I. Anal. Biochem. 16, 395 (1966).
8. Salas, M., Vinuela, E. & Sols, A. J. Biol. Chem. 238, 3535 (1963).
9. Beers, R. F., Jr. & Sizer, I. W. J. Biol. Chem. 195, 133 (1952).
10. Pitot, H. C. & Pries, N. Anal. Biochem. 9, 454 (1964).
11. Bresnick, E., Mayfield, E. D., Jr. & Mosse, H. Mol. Pharmacol. 4, 173 (1968).
12. Ciotti, M. M. & Kaplan, N. O. in Methods in Enzymology (S. P. Colowick & N. O. Kaplan, eds.) Vol. III, 890 (1957).
13. Lowry, O. H., Rosebrough. N. J., Farr, A. L. & Randall, R. J. J. Biol. Chem. 193, 265 (1951).
14. Kunitz, M. J. Gen. Physiol. 30, 291 (1947).
15. Rosen, H. Arch. Biochem. Biophys. 67, 10 (1957).
16. Schimke, R. T. & Doyle, D. Ann. Rev. Biochem. 39, 929 (1970).
17. Price, V. E., Sterling, W. R., Tarantola, V. A., Hartley, R. W., Jr. & Rechcigl, M., Jr. J. Biol. Chem. 237, 3468 (1962).
18. Greenbaum, A. L., Gumaa, K. A. & McLean, P. Arch. Biochem. Biophys. 143, 617 (1971).
19. Johnson, R. W. & Kenney, F. T. J. Biol. Chem. 248, 4528 (1973).

20. Segal, H. L., Matsuzawa, T., Haider, M. & Abraham, G. J. Biochem. Biophys. Res. Commun. 36, 764 (1969).

21. Li, J. B. & Knox, W. E. J. Biol. Chem. 247, 7550, (1972).

22. Haider, M. & Segal, H. L. Arch. Biochem. Biophys. 148, 228 (1972).

23. Dice, J. F., Dehlinger, P. J. & Schimke, R. T. J. Biol. Chem. 248, 4220 (1973).

24. Barman, T. E. (ed.) Enzyme Handbook, Springer-Verlag, New York (1969).

25. Sober, H. A. (ed.) Handbook of Biochemistry, 2nd edition, The Chemical Rubber Co., Cleveland, Ohio (1970).

26. Inoue, H., Kasper, C. B. & Pitot, H. C. J. Biol. Chem. 246, 2626 (1971).

TURNOVER OF IODINATED PLASMA MEMBRANE PROTEINS OF HEPATOMA TISSUE CULTURE CELLS

John Tweto and Darrell Doyle

Department of Molecular Biology
Roswell Park Memorial Institute
Buffalo, New York 14203

Summary

Rat liver hepatoma tissue culture (HTC) cells have been labeled with ^{125}I by a lactoperoxidase catalyzed reaction. The label is confined to the plasma membrane and is present as monoiodotyrosine in the proteins of the plasma membrane. Between 10 and 15 polypeptides in the membrane have tyrosine residues accessible to the lactoperoxidase probe. These polypeptides turn over as judged by the release of monoiodotyrosine into the suspension medium. Proteolytic hydrolysis of the total membrane fraction, followed by fingerprinting reveals a characteristic pattern of iodinated peptides. These peptides are being assigned to specific membrane proteins with the ultimate goal of examining in detail the organization and biogenesis of the proteins of the limiting cell membrane.

For the past several years, we have been examining the relative roles of synthesis and degradation in the regulation of protein level in liver cells and subcellular organelles (1-6). These types of studies are dependent on radioisotopic labeling procedures usually employing ^{3}H or ^{14}C amino acids to label the bulk of cell proteins, followed by immunological or classical purification techniques to isolate the organelle or enzyme of interest. Recently, we have become involved in an attempt to follow the pathway of degradation of either a specific liver protein or

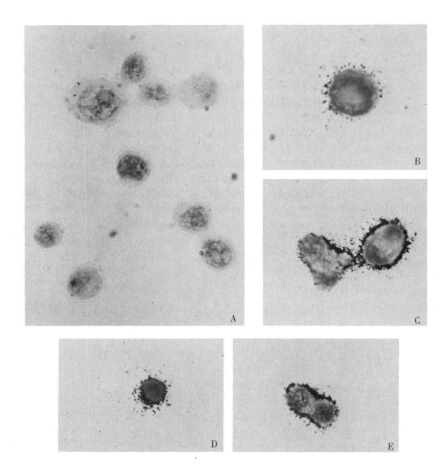

Figure 1: HTC cells were iodinated using an H_2O_2
generating system (8). The cells were air dried
on a microscope slide and fixed in methanol. The
slides were washed with water, dried and coated
with Kodak NTB-3 liquid emulsion. (A) Control in
which lactoperoxidase was omitted. (B) Cell after
30 min iodination. (C, D, E) Cells after 60 min
iodination.

groups of proteins within an organized cell structure. Radioisotopic labeling procedures are also required for this type of study but methods which label bulk cell protein cannot be used. Ideally, one would like to be able to label a single enzyme or cell organelle in situ without affecting either cell viability, normal cell metabolism or the turnover of the structure or enzyme that has been specifically labeled. The cell organelle that is most amenable to study in this respect is the plasma membrane because it is accessible to labeling from the outside by methods which should not label other cellular constituents (7-9). We are using lactoperoxidase catalyzed iodination with $Na^{125}I$ as a probe to study the biogenesis of the plasma membrane of Hepatoma tissue culture (HTC) cells. This cell line was chosen for study because it was derived originally from a rat hepatic tumor. Liver has been the organ of choice for most protein turnover studies and HTC cells would be expected to use the same or similar degradative mechanisms as the hepatocyte. Indeed, studies on the turnover of a characteristic liver enzyme, tyrosine aminotransferase, indicate that the regulation of this protein in HTC cells is similar to that in rat liver (10-12). Further, HTC cells have been well characterized as to growth, karyotype, and morphology, and these cells are responsive to various hormonal and physiological effectors.

HTC cells can be labeled to high specific activity with ^{125}I in the presence of lactoperoxidase and H_2O_2 or an H_2O_2 generating system composed of glucose oxidase and glucose (7-9). As shown in Table I after iodination the label is present predominantly in a sedimentable cell fraction, presumably the plasma membrane. The specific activity of proteins in this fraction is at least 25 times that of the soluble proteins. Radioautographs of iodinated cells shown in Fig. 1 further demonstrate that the label is associated almost exclusively with the cell surface.

The lactoperoxidase catalyzed iodination labels only the proteins of the plasma membrane; enzymatic hydrolysis with pronase and pancreatin of a membrane

297

TABLE I.

Distribution of ^{125}I-Radioactivity in HTC Cells

Cell Fraction	Protein	^{125}I-Radioactivity	Specific Activity
	mg/5 x 10^6 cells	DPM x 10^{-5}/5 x 10^6 cells	DPM/mg x 10^{-5} protein
Homogenate	0.82	5.7	6.9
Supernatant	0.76	0.85	1.1
Pellet	0.12	3.5	29.2

TABLE II.

Labeling of HTC Cells with ^{125}I

Conditions of Labeling	^{125}I Incorporated
	DPM x 10^{-5}/5 x 10^6 Cells
1. HTC Cells + ^{125}I + LP + H_2O_2	9.5
2. HTC Cells + ^{125}I	0.5
3. (HTC Cells + Trypsin) + ^{125}I + LP + H_2O_2	2.9
4. HTC Cells + Collagenase-hyaluronidase + ^{125}I + LP + H_2O_2	7.7
5. (HTC Cells + ^{125}I + LP + H_2O_2) + Trypsin	2.7

298

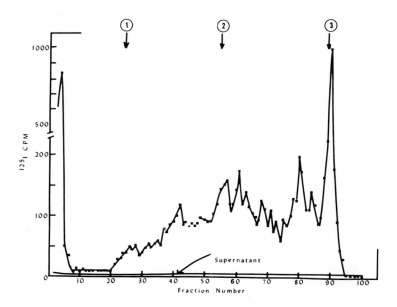

Figure 3:   HTC cells were iodinated with ^{125}I and
separated into a pellet and a soluble fraction.
The proteins in each fraction were dissociated
by heating at 100° in the presence of 1% SDS and
1% 2-mercaptoethanol.   The dissociated polypeptides
were separated by SDS-acrylamide gel electrophoresis (14).   Arrows indicate approximate molecular weights: (1) 130,000; (2) 68,000; (3) 12,000.

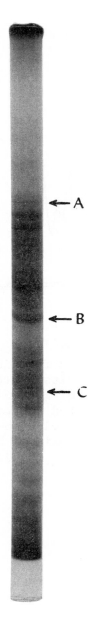

Figure 2: SDS-Polyacrylamide electrophoresis of the polypeptides from HTC cell plasma membranes. Approximate molecular weights are indicated by the arrows: (A) 68,000 daltons, (B) 45,000 daltons, (C) 25,000 daltons.

fraction isolated from HTC cells releases more than 99% of the incorporated label as monoiodotyrosine. By diluting the radioactive iodide with unlabeled iodide, it is possible to titrate the sites present on the cells, and such analysis shows approximately 10^7 sites per cell. Furthermore, iodination does not effect the viability of the cells as judged by trypan blue exclusion and iodinated cells grow normally.

To determine the distribution of incorporated iodide, a plasma membrane fraction from HTC cells was prepared by the latex bead method of Charalampons, et al. (13). The membrane was dissociated in SDS and 2-mercaptoethanol and the polypeptides were separated by SDS-polyacrylamide gel electrophoresis (14). As shown in Fig. 2, the polypeptide composition of the HTC cell membrane is rather complex. But, as shown by the ^{125}I-radioactivity profile (Fig. 3) only 10-15 of the membrane proteins have tyrosine residues that are accessible to the lactoperoxidase probe. No labeled proteins are present in the soluble fraction of the cell. Radioautographs of SDS-polyacrylamide gels also reveal 10-15 labeled proteins from the plasma membrane. Treatment of the HTC cell with trypsin before iodination reduces the amount of iodide incorporated by about 70% while treatment of the cell with trypsin after iodination removes the same amount of label (Table II). All of the preceding experiments indicate that only proteins of the limiting cell membrane are labeled by the lactoperoxidase probe.

The experiment presented in Fig. 4 and Table III was designed to assess the effect of plasma membrane iodination on total protein turnover in HTC cells and to determine if iodinated plasma membrane proteins turn over.

HTC cells were grown for several generations in the presence of ^{14}C tyrosine. When the specific radioactivity of cell protein reached a maximum, the cells were collected and washed free of labeled tyrosine. The cells then were iodinated with sufficient unlabeled iodide to saturate the available sites. Cells were incubated at 37° or 4° and aliquots were removed at the

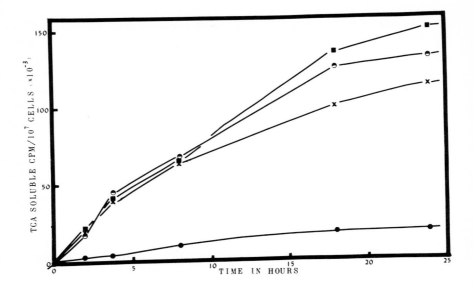

Figure 4: HTC cells were grown in suspension culture
for three generations in medium containing ^{14}C-
tyrosine (U). The cells were collected, washed
with Earles salt solution, and iodinated with
unlabeled KI using lactoperoxidase and the H_2O_2
generating system. Total TCA insoluble radioactivity
was determined with a portion of the cells. The TCA
insoluble residue was then hydrolyzed with pronase
and pancreatin and ^{14}C-monoiodotyrosine was separated from ^{14}C-tyrosine by thin layer chromatography.
There were 1.4×10^6 cells/ml. One culture contained
latex particles throughout the incubation. Aliquots
were removed at the times indicated and total TCA
soluble radioactivity determined. The radioactivity
in the TCA soluble fraction as monoiodotyrosine was
assayed after separation by thin layer chromatography.
These results are presented in Table III.

0—0 incubation at 4°.
X—X incubation at 37° with latex beads
     incubation at 37°
0—0 incubation at 37° plus iodination.

TABLE III.

Release of ^{14}C-Monoiodotyrosine from HTC Cells

Time of Incubation (Hours)	Experimental Conditions	^{14}C-CPM as Monoiodotyrosine/10^7 Cells
0	HTC Cells, 37°	200
	HTC Cells + Latex Particles, 37°	150
8	HTC Cells, 37°	700
	HTC Cells + Latex Particles, 37°	7920
18	HTC Cells, 37°	7000
	HTC Cells + Latex Particles	9200

Experimental details for this table are given in the legend to Figure 4.

TABLE IV.

The Effect of Iodination on Protein Turnover
As Measured by a Double Isotope Procedure

	CELL FRACTION (10^5 Cells)					
	Membrane			Soluble		
Conditions	DPM H^3	DPM ^{14}C	^{3}H:^{14}C	DPM ^{3}H	DPM ^{14}C	^{3}H:^{14}C
Iodinated	34,400	9,400	3.66	34,400	9,800	3.51
Control	55,000	14,000	3.93	36,800	9,200	4.00

Duplicate cultures of washed HTC cells were suspended in media without serum or tyrosine. One culture was iodinated using the glucose oxidase system to generate H_2O_2 but 1.1 nanomoles of unlabeled KI was used in place of ^{125}I. KI was not added to the other culture which served as a control. After stirring for 40 minutes, each culture was washed, resuspended in growth media without serum, and divided into two. To each of the four cultures 10 µCi of ^{14}C leucine (U) was added. The cultures were stirred for one hour at 37°. They were then washed, resuspended in 3 ml of growth media without serum but containing 0.25% BSA, and incubated for 21 hours at 37°C. At this time 50 µC of ^{3}H-leucine (4,5^{3}H) was added and the cells were stirred for an additional hour. The cells were collected, washed, and frozen and thawed three times. The extracts were separated into a soluble and a sedimentable fraction. The TCA insoluble material in each sample was dissolved in Protosol (New England Nuclear), counted, and the ^{3}H and ^{14}C values were calculated. Data from duplicate cultures were averaged.

times indicated. Both total TCA soluble radioactivity and radioactivity as ^{14}C-monoiodotyrosine were determined. Lactoperoxidase catalyzed iodination converts 5% of the TCA insoluble radioactivity from tyrosine to monoiodotyrisine. The iodinated plasma membrane proteins turn over with time. As expected, protein degradation in these cells is temperature dependent.

The addition of polystyrene latex beads to the medium promotes interiorization of large portions of the plasma membrane as a result of phagocytosis (15). The phagosome bodies undergo fusion within the cell with lysosomes and the contents are digested. As shown in Table III in the presence of the latex beads the cell turns over increased amounts of plasma membrane proteins releasing large amounts of iodotyrosine.

In similar experiments we have monitored the release of TCA soluble radioactivity from HTC cells labeled with ^{125}I. The results are consistent with those presented in Fig. 4 and Table III but are complicated by the fact that lactoperoxidase for some reason promotes the retention of iodide by these cells and a large percentage of the released radioactivity is in the form of iodide. As also shown in Fig. 4, extensive iodination does not appreciably effect the turnover of total cell protein as far as can be judged by the release of tyrosine into the medium. This way of measuring turnover is rather insensitive, however, since the release of amino acids is a step quite far removed from the presumed rate limiting step in protein degradation.

A double isotope procedure (16) was used to assess the effect of iodination on the rate constant of degradation of both soluble protein and membrane protein, the results of which are presented in Table IV. The difference of the isotope ratios in the two experiments suggest a slight effect on total protein turnover. However, this difference is within the limits of experimental error and is probably not significant. Since the isotope ratios in this type of experiment are directly proportional to the rate constants of degradation (3), this experiment suggests

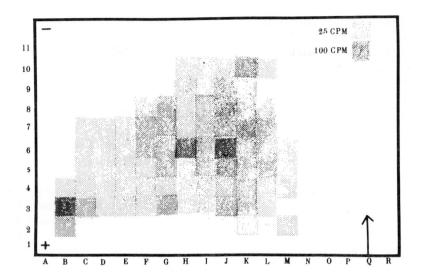

Figure 5: Thin layer electrophoresis and chromatography of the ^{125}I peptides released from a
membrane fraction of HTC cells by trypsin. The
arrow indicates the distance migrated by the
solvent front. Conditions for hydrolysis, chromatography and electrophoresis are given in (5).
Iodinated peptides were located by cutting the
silica gel sheet into 1 cm squares and counting
in a scintillation spectrometer.

that iodination has little or no effect on total protein turnover. The apparent half-life for total cell
protein in these experiments is 28 hours.

The evidence presented thus far shows that it is
feasible to use lactoperoxidase catalyzed iodination
of HTC cells as a probe for studying the turnover of
plasma membrane proteins. We now wish to extend these
experiments to examine the organization of the iodinated proteins in the membrane; to examine certain
aspects of plasma membrane biogenesis, particularly
the problem of whether there exists in the cell a
pool of membrane precursor proteins as has been suggested by others (17,18); to determine if turnover
of the membrane proteins occurs in an organized manner;
to determine whether there is heterogeneity in turnover rates among the membrane proteins (19); to isolate if possible intermediates in the degradation of
the membrane proteins, and finally, to attempt to
assign functions to some of the proteins using blocking reactions prior to iodination.

Our ability to do these studies is dependent on a
method of identifying the iodinated membrane proteins
other than by their mobility in acrylamide gels. Two
of the most sensitive methods of characterizing proteins are by amino acid sequencing or by analyzing
peptides released by proteolytic hydrolysis. Figure
5 is a representation of the peptides containing [125]I
which have been released by trypsin from a plasma
membrane fraction of HTC cells. Several distinct
peptides are apparent. We are now in the process of
assigning these peptides to the different iodinated
membrane proteins separated by SDS-acrylamide electrophoresis. Thus far, only one tryptic peptide has been
assigned to a specific membrane protein. When the
assignment of specific peptides to specific membrane
proteins is complete, we believe that the system described in this report may be able to provide significant information on the organization, biogenesis,
and function of specific proteins in the limiting
membrane of these cells.

Acknowledgement

Our work is supported by the U. S. Public Health Service through grants HD08410 and GM19521. We thank them. We also thank Eliza Friedman for technical assistance and Dr. Tom Gelehrter for supplying the cells, and Christina Doyle for help in preparing Fig. 5.

References

1. Tweto, J., Liberati, M. & Larrabee, A. R. J. Biol. Chem. 246, 2468 (1971).
2. Tweto, J. & Larrabee, A. R. J. Biol. Chem. 246, 4900 (1972).
3. Glass, R. D. & Doyle, D. J. Biol. Chem. 247, 5234 (1972).
4. Schimke, R. T. & Doyle, D. Ann. Rev. Biochem. 39, 929 (1970).
5. Doyle, D. J. Biol. Chem. 246, 4965 (1971).
6. Glass, R. D. & Doyle, D. Science 176, 180 (1972).
7. Phillips, D. R. & Morrison, M. Biochemistry 10, 1766 (1971).
8. Hubbard, A. L. & Cohn, Z. A. J. Cell Biol. 55, 390 (1972).
9. Nachman, R. L., Hubbard, A. & Ferris, B. J. Biol. Chem. 248, 2928 (1973).
10. Tomkins, G. M., Gelehrter, T. D., Granner, D., Martin, D., Jr., Samuels, H. H., & Thompson, E. B. Science 166, 1474 (1969).
11. Hershko, A. & Tomkins, G. M. J. Biol. Chem. 246, 710 (1971).
12. Lee, K. & Kenney, F. T. J. Biol. Chem. 246, 7595 (1971).
13. Charalampous, F. C., Gonatas, N. K. & Melbourne, A. D. J. Cell Biol. 59, 421 (1973).
14. Laemmli, U. K. Nature 227, 680 (1970).
15. Hubbard, A. L., Cohn, Z. A. J. Cell Biol. 59, 152a (1973).
16. Arias, I. M., Doyle, D. & Schimke, R. T. J. Biol. Chem. 244, 3303 (1969).

17. Ray, T. K., Lieberman, I. & Lansing, A. I.
    Biochem. Biophys. Res. Commun. 31, 54 (1968).
18. Barancik-Cohen, L. & Lieberman, I. Biochem.
    Biophys. Res. Commun. 44, 1084 (1971).
19. Dehlinger, P. J. & Schimke, R. T. J. Biol. Chem.
    246, 2574 (1971).

Specific Problems in Turnover
of Proteins

PROTEIN DEGRADATION IN NORMAL, TRANSFORMED, AND SENESCENT HUMAN FIBROBLASTS

Matthews O. Bradley and Robert T. Schimke

Department of Biological Sciences
Stanford University
Stanford, California 94305

Cellular senescence and malignant transformation may result from either specific genetic action or from stochastic errors of molecular replication and structure. Error theories posit primary damage to either DNA, RNA, lipid, or protein. Because the cell manufactures all of its own components, an inaccurate synthetic machinery would have to be repaired or an increased error frequency would destroy the cell. For example, decreased fidelity of DNA synthesis would increase the mutation frequency which could produce malignant variation or cell death. Likewise, decreased fidelity of protein synthesis could produce an "error catastrophe" of the sort envisaged by Orgel (1,2). Since DNA, RNA, and protein synthesis are interdependent, a replicating error in one of them should inevitably lead to errors in the others.

Mechanisms of DNA repair are well known; protein repair, however, is unknown. Protein degradation may provide the functional equivalent of repair by selectively eliminating those proteins with altered structure. Support for this concept comes from recent evidence that primary structural alterations or amino acid analog substitutions increase the rate of a protein's degradation in both cell-free and intact systems (3-7). The total error frequency during protein synthesis may amount to 3×10^{-4} errors per amino acid residue (8); this means that approximately 15% of all

50,000 dalton proteins will have one amino acid mis-
incorporation. Selective degradation of such proteins
may be necessary for cell survival. Transitions from
normalcy to malignancy or senescence could result from
an altered capacity of cells to degrade abnormal proteins generated through transcriptional and translational errors in protein synthesis.

This paper attempts to define what role protein
degradation plays in embryonic, senescent, and transformed cells. For these studies, we have used the
normal human embryonic fibroblast strain WI-38 (9,10),
in its active (phase II) and senescent (phase III)
growth phases, and in a malignant cell line, VA-13,
derived from WI-38 by SV-40 virus transformation (11).
This system has the advantage of being well-defined
since both senescent and malignant cells arise from
the same normal fibroblast. We describe different
methods for measuring protein degradation in cultured
cells and compare rates of degradation in embryonic,
senescent, and malignant cells.

Materials and Methods

WI-38 cells and their SV-40 transformed variant,
VA-13, were serially subcultured in 75 cm^2 growth
area tissue culture flasks or in 32 oz glass prescrip-
tion bottles in Eagle's Basal Medium (GIBCO, powdered
BME) with 10% calf serum, 28 mM Hepes, 1 mM L-gluta-
mine, and 50 μg/ml aureomycin. All cells were free of
mycoplasma contamination. The young (phase II) WI-38
cells had undergone no more than 28 population doub-
lings in vitro. Senescent (phase III) WI-38 cells were
defined by: their granular and uneven microscopic
appearance, their inability to form confluent monolayers, and their ultimate loss of mitotic activity.

Protein degradation was measured in cells grown in
either 25 cm^2 growth area plastic tissue culture flasks
or in glass scintillation vials. Isotopic leucine
(L-leucine-4,5-^{3}H and U-^{14}C) was added directly to
complete medium.

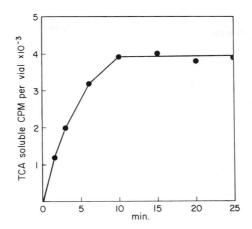

Figure 1A: Leucine flux in confluent monolayers of WI-38. ^{3}H-leucine was added in series to duplicate cultures in glass scintillation vials. Uptake was stopped by rapidly cooling and washing the cultures 3 times with 5 ml of ice-cold BME. After aspirating off the last of the wash, TCA (5%, 1 ml, ice-cold) was added for 2 hr. TCA soluble radioactivity taken up by the monolayers is plotted on the ordinate as a function of time after isotope addition.

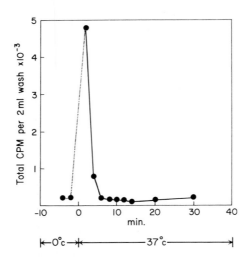

Figure 1B: Monolayer cultures in glass scintillation
vials were labeled with ^{3}H-leucine for either 15
minutes or 50 hours. After labeling, the vials
were chilled and washed 10 times with ice-cold BME
until the wash radioactivity was negligible. Then
the vials were reincubated at 37°C in BME containing 10% calf serum; every 2 minutes the medium was
removed and another 2 ml of medium added. The
radioactivity in each wash is plotted as a function
of time. The kinetics of label efflux are the same,
no matter whether the cells were labeled for 15
minutes or 50 hours. At the end of each experiment,
5% TCA was added to determine the amount of TCA
soluble radioactivity remaining in the cultures.

Cells pulsed for 15 minutes contained 4% of the
initial TCA-soluble label, while cells labeled
for 50 hours contained 25% of the initial TCA-soluble
label.

Results

Leucine Flux. The rate of uptake and loss of free
^{3}H-leucine by confluent monolayers of WI-38 was determined as shown in Fig. 1. TCA-soluble leucine radioactivity reached a maximum value within 7 minutes after
addition of isotope (Fig. 1a). The rate of loss of
free ^{3}H-leucine from internal pools was determined in
cells that had been labeled for either 15 minutes or
50 hours. Free leucine was lost by the internal pools
within 5-7 minutes in both experiments (Fig. 1b). Fifteen minutes after washing began, 4% of the initial
TCA-soluble radioactivity remained within pulse-labeled
cells while 25% remained within continuously labeled
cells. In the latter case, the amount of TCA-soluble
radioactivity was 0.25% of the total protein radioactivity. It is not known whether this retained radioactivity represents a contamination by TCA-soluble protein, a non-exchangeable leucine pool, or a steady-
state flux through internal pools due to protein breakdown and leucine efflux.

Measurements of Protein Degradation. Measurements
of the decay of pre-labeled proteins are often complicated by the reutilization of isotopic precursor amino
acids. This problem can be overcome by measuring the
rate of approach of cellular protein to a constant isotopic specific activity (12). The rate of approach is
dependent upon the rate of protein degradation so long
as the cells are in a steady-state, the rate of protein
synthesis is constant, and the specific activity of the
precursor pools is constant.

Using this approach to equilibrium method, we have
determined that the mean half-life of protein in young,
senescent, and transformed WI-38 cells is 20 hours
(Table I). The following quantities were approximately
constant during these experiments: the protein mass
per culture, the amount of TCA-soluble radioactivity
in the intracellular pools, and the amount of ^{14}C-
leucine incorporated into TCA-precipitable material
during a one-hour pulse. The constancy of these
measurements implies that the cultures were in a steady
state during these experiments.

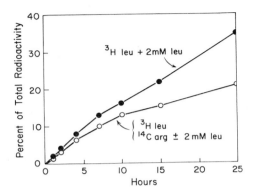

Figure 2: Effect of excess leucine on release of TCA-soluble radioactivity into the medium. WI-38 confluent monolayers were labeled with ^{3}H-leucine and ^{14}C arginine; then they were washed and reincubated in normal medium or medium supplemented with 2 mM leucine. Aliquots (100 λ from 6 ml total) of the medium were removed during the experiment and assayed for radioactivity.

TABLE I.

Method	$\dagger$, Phase II WI-38	$\dagger$, Early Phase III WI-38	$\dagger$, Late Phase III WI-38	$\dagger$, VA-13
Approach to Equilibrium	21	20	–	20
Intermittent Perfusion 25 min Labeling	6	3	3	6
Intermittent Perfusion 40 hr Labeling	37	37	29	37

Mean half-lives of protein in WI-38 and VA-13 cells as determined by different methods. The half-life, $\dagger$, is defined as :

$$\dagger = \frac{\ln 2}{k}$$

where k is the rate constant for the protein fraction degraded per hour.

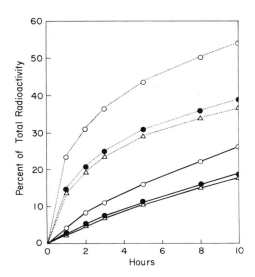

Figure 3: Kinetics of protein degradation in Phase
II, Phase III and SV-40 transformed WI-38 cells.
Monolayer cultures were prelabeled for 40 hours
with ^{14}C-leucine, washed for 2 hours, and then
relabeled for 25 minutes with ^{3}H-leucine. The
kinetics of TCA-soluble isotope release were determined by the intermittent perfusion method described
in the text. Terminal Phase III WI-38 (0); Phase II
WI38 (0); SV-40 WI-38 (△). Dotted lines: 25 minute,
^{3}H leucine. Solid lines: 40 hour, ^{14}C-leucine.

(14,15) have noted that reutilization can obscure accurate determinations of protein half-life in cell cultures.

Since the approach to equilibrium method is experimentally limited because of its relative insensitivity and steady state assumptions, we attempted to minimize the amount of reutilization occurring in radioactive decay measurements of protein degradation. The intermittent perfusion method (Table I) generates much shorter values for protein half-lives (35 hours) than does the standard aliquot removal method (90 hours). Reutilization has been greatly reduced by probably not completely eliminated since protein half-lives after a 40-hour continuous labeling are still somewhat longer than values determined by the approach to equilibrium method and also since some radioactivity may not be removed from the long-labeled pools (Fig. 1b). On the other hand, reutilization is not likely to effect measurements of rapidly turning over protein since pulse-labeled pools can be rapidly emptied of all isotope (Fig. 1b). For these reasons, we assume in the remaining discussion that our results are not due to differential reutilization of leucine.

The intermittent perfusion method shows that the rate of protein degradation in senescent (phase III) WI-38 cells is greater than the rate in young (phase II) cultures (Table I). The first differences occur in early phase III; pulse-labeled protein is degraded more rapidly while long-labeled proteins are degraded at the same rates. By the end of phase III, both short and long-lived proteins are being degraded faster. Protein degradation in the transformed VA-13 cells is similar to that in young WI-38 cells. All these results are consistent with observations that residual lysozymes and lysosomal enzymes increase in phase III cultures (16-19).

These findings support the protein-error theory of Orgel (1,2), which postulates that errors in protein synthesis become self-propagating. As pointed out in the introduction, the protein degradative system may function in a "quality control" capacity by preferentially degrading error-containing protein. If the

The approach to equilibrium method is experimentally limited because of its steady-state assumptions.
For this reason, we tested various methods for measuring the decay of prelabeled protein. We first determined the effect of higher leucine concentrations in
the medium on the rate of release of leucine from prelabeled cells (Fig. 2). WI-38 cultures were pre-labeled
for hours with ^{3}H-leucine and ^{14}C arginine; then they
were washed and reincubated either in normal medium
or in medium supplemented with 2 mM leucine. Aliquots
(100 µl from 6 ml total) of the medium were removed
and assayed for radioactivity. The mean half-life of
protein labeled with ^{3}H-leucine and incubated in normal medium was 87 hours while that incubated in medium
supplemented with 2 mM leucine was 57 hours. The half-
life of protein labeled with ^{14}C-arginine was not
altered by the additional leucine. This experiment
indicates that reutilization of isotopic precursor
occurs in cell monolayers since increasing the leucine
concentration of the medium significantly reduces the
apparent protein half-life.

Leucine fluxes in and out of the cell occur extremely
rapidly as shown in Fig. 1. The rate of uptake is equal
to the rate of loss as one would expect in steady-state
conditions. We have attempted to create a more efficient trap for intracellular isotopic leucine by ex-
ploiting this flux. We wash prelabeled cells 10 times
with medium supplemented with 2 mM leucine in order to
empty the internal pools of isotopic leucine as much
as possible. The cultures are incubated in a shaking
water bath; every hour for the first 3 hours and every
2-3 hours thereafter, the medium was completely removed
and replaced with new medium. Aliquots of each medium
change were counted in a water-miscible scintillation
fluid. No TCA-precipitable radioactivity was recovered
in the medium. This procedure generates values for
protein half-lives of approximately 25 to 40 hours for
young, confluent WI-38 cells isotopically labeled for
40 hours (Table I). These half-lives are significantly
less than values obtained by aliquot removal and are
similar to values obtained by the approach to equilibrium

method. We conclude that some reutilization may still occur with this intermittent perfusion method; however, its magnitude must be small since another method, not subject to reutilization, produces similar data.

We have re-examined protein degradation in young, senescent, and transformed WI-38 cells by the perfusion method. This method enables us to study both rapidly and slowly turning over proteins by labeling cultures with different isotopes for short and long periods. The protocol was to first label stationary phase cultures with 0.25 μci/ml of ^{14}C-leucine for 40 hours. Then the cells were washed 4 times and reincubated in fresh medium containing 2 mM unlabeled leucine. The ^{14}C-protein was allowed to decay for 2 hours; this medium was discarded and the cells were labeled again with 40 μci/ml of ^{3}H-leucine for 25 minutes. After this labeling regime, the cultures were handled as described above for the perfusion method. Such a protocol will label long-lived proteins with ^{14}C-leucine and short-lived proteins with ^{3}H-leucine.

Table I shows that short-lived, but not long-lived, protein is degraded at faster rates in WI-38 cells at the beginning of senescence (phase III). At the very end of phase III, however, both short-lived and long-lived proteins turn over faster than do proteins in young, phase II cells. The rates of degradation in the transformed derivative, VA-13, are the same as those of phase II WI-38 cells.

Discussion

Reutilization biases measurements of protein half-lives towards larger values when they are determined by the decay of prelabeled protein in monolayer cell cultures (Fig. 2). The approach to equilibrium method, theoretically at least, is not subject to reutilization; protein half-lives determined by this method are approximately 20 hours. This value is much faster than previous estimates of protein degradation in cell culture (13) which were about 1% per hour (a half-life of 69 hours). Whether these discrepancies are due solely to reutilization is not known, although other authors error frequency of protein synthesis increases in phase III as postulated by Orgel, then preferential degradation of error-containing protein would increase the overall rate of protein degradation as we have demonstrated. Since error-containing protein should be rapidly degradable, it is reasonable that increased pulse-labeled protein degradation should be detectable first in early phase III. At the end of phase III more of the total protein may contain errors, so that the rate of long-labeled protein degradation increases also. Terminal phase III would then result from a functional failure of the protein degradative system; due either to synthesis of an overwhelming amount of error-containing protein that cannot be degraded rapidly engouth or to a defective degradative system that has lost its capacity to select "abnormal" protein, or a combination of the two possibilities.

This work suggests that one of the important functions of intracellular protein degradation may be to reduce the amount of error-containing protein, thereby ensuring cellular homeostasis and survival. If this is true, then senescent or malignant alterations may be accompanied by changes in the functional capacity of cells to recognize and degrade error-containing protein.

References

1. Orgel, L. E.   Proc. Nat. Acad. Sci. USA 49, 517 (1963).
2. Orgel, L. E.   Proc. Nat. Acad. Sci. USA 67, 1476 (1970).
3. Pine, M. J.   J. Bacteriol. 93, 1527 (1967).
4. Goldschmidt, R.   Nature 228, 1151 (1970).
5. Platt, T., Miller, J. & Weber, K.   Nature 228, 1154 (1970).
6. Goldberg, A. L.   Proc. Nat. Acad. Sci. USA 69, 422 (1972).
7. Goldberg, A. L.   Proc. Nat. Acad. Sci. USA 69, 2640 (1972).
8. Loftfield, R. B.   Biochem. J. 89, 82 (1963).

9. Hayflick, L. & Moorhead, P. S. Exp. Cell Res.
      25, 585 (1961).
10. Hayflick, L. Exp. Cell Res. 37, 614 (1965).
11. Girardi, A. J., Jensen, F. C. & Koprowski, H.
      J. Cell Comp. Physiol. 65, 69 (1965).
12. Schimke, R. T. Mammalian Protein Metabolism
      (H. N. Munro, ed.), New York, Academic Press,
      p. 177 (1970).
13. Eagle, H., Piez, K. A., Fleischman, R. & Oyama,
      V. I. J. Biol. Chem. 234, 592 (1959).
14. Klevecz, R. Biochem. Biophys. Res. Commun. 43,
      76 (1971).
15. Righetti, P., Little, E. P. & Wolf, G. J.Biol.
      Chem. 246, 5724 (1971).
16. Cristofalo, V. J., Parris, N. & Kritchevsky, D.
      J. Cell Physiol. 69, 263 (1967).
17. Brock, M. A. & Hay, R. J. J. Ultrastruct. Res.
      36, 291 (1971).
18. Lipetz, J. & Cristofalo, V. J. J. Ultrastruct.
      Res. 39, 43 (1972).
19. Brunk, U., Ericsson, J. L. E., Ponten, J. &
      Westermark, B. Exptl. Cell Res. 79, 1 (1973).

TURNOVER OF MICROSOMAL ENZYMES IN RAT LIVER

Tsuneo Omura

Department of Biology
Faculty of Science, Kyushu University
Fukuoka, Japan

Most presentations at this symposium are concerned with the turnover of soluble enzyme proteins which are present in the cytoplasm of cells. The protein components of various intracellular membranes also turn over at least as rapidly as the soluble proteins in the same cell, and the characteristic compositions of these membranes are maintained by the dynamic equilibrium between the degradation and new supply of their components. I should like to discuss in this paper the turnover of microsomal membrane-bound enzyme proteins which constitute the integral part of the membrane structure. The first topic to be discussed is the independent turnover of membrane constituents.

Since morphological observations by electron-microscope frequently show the engulfment of endoplasmic reticulum membranes or mitochondrial particles by lysosomes in the liver cells, there is a concept that these membranes are degraded as a whole. If such is the case, all protein constituents of a given membrane should have the identical turnover rate. However, the biochemical evidence provided by recent turnover studies on microsomal membrane components (1,2,3) is not consistent with such a concept.

Many kinds of enzymes are present in the microsomes of rat liver, but the components of the microsomal NADH-linked and NADPH-linked electron-transport chains seem to be most suitable for studying the independent turnover of microsomal membrane proteins because the

interacting components of an electron-transport chain
should be present in the same portion of the membrane.
NADH-cytochrome b_5 reductase and cytochrome b_5 constitute the main compounds of the NADH-linked electron-
transport chain of microsomes. NADPH-cytochrome c
reductase and cytochrome P-450 are intimately associated with each other in the transfer of electrons
for oxygenation reactions from NADPH. There is also
strong evidence for the cross-reactions between these
two electron-transport chains in intact microsomal
membrane, so the molecules of these two pairs of redox
enzymes must be present together in the membrane.

None of these four enzymes is the predominant component of the microsomal membrane (Table I), but of
them, cytochrome b_5, NADH-cytochrome b_5 reductase,
and NADPH-cytochrome c reductase may be readily purified starting from small amounts of microsomes. They
can be easily and relatively specifically solubilized
from microsomes by suitable protease treatments. Cytochrome b_5 and NADPH-cytochrome c reductase can be
solubilized by trypsin digestion (1). NADH-cytochrome
b_5 reductase cannot be solubilized by trypsin treatment, but specifically solubilized by the digestion by
lysosomal extracts (4). Although the solubilized enzymes are the proteolytic fragments of the membrane-
bound native molecules (5), the ease of purification
of protease-solubilized enzymes made them much more
suitable for turnover studies than their native counterparts. The easy solubilization of these microsomal
enzymes by protease treatments suggests their outside
localization in the microsomal vesicles (6), which has
also been confirmed by immunochemical techniques using
enzyme-specific antibodies (Table I). We have also
studied the turnover of two other microsomal enzymes,
carboxy esterase and nucleoside diphosphatase, which
are both present on the inside surface of the vesicles
(7,8)(Table I).

Figure 1 shows a typical example of our turnover
studies on these enzymes. After the in vivo labeling
by the intravenous injection of radioactive leucine
into rats, the three enzymes were purified from the

TABLE I.

Content of Enzymes in Rat Liver Microsomes

Enzyme	Content (% of total protein)	Sideness in vesicle
Cytochrome b_5	1.0	outside
NADH-cytochrome b_5 reductase	0.2	outside
Cytochrome P-450	5.0	?
NADPH-cytochrome c reductase	0.5	outside
Carboxyesterase	2.0	inside
Nucleoside diphosphatase	0.5	inside

TABLE II.

Half-lives of Microsomal Enzymes in Rat Liver

Enzyme	Half-life (hr)	Reference
Cytochrome b_5	100	(18)
NADH-cytochrome b_5 reductase	140	(9)
NADPH-cytochrome c reductase	70	(18)
Nucleoside diphosphatase	30	(8)
Carboxyesterase	95	(10)
HMG-CoA reductase	4	(11)
NAD glycohydrolase	430	(12)

325

liver microsomes of the same animals killed at the
time points as shown in the Figure, and the loss of
radioactivity from the enzyme proteins was followed.
Their turnover rates were clearly different.

Table II summarizes the results thus obtained.
These microsomal enzymes, "outside-located" enzymes
as well as "inside-located" ones, have their own independent turnover rates. Even NADH-cytochrome b_5 reductase and cytochrome b_5, which should be present
together in the membrane interacting in the transfer
of electrons from NADH to cytochrome b_5, showed different turnover rates. Two more microsomal enzymes
with very different half-lives, hydroxymethylglutaryl
coenzyme A reductase and NAD glycohydrolase, are also
included in Table II for comparison. As is clearly
seen, some microsomal membrane enzymes have very short
half-lives, while some others have much longer half-
lives. These various kinds of enzymes, which are
present in the same membrane as the integral components of the membrane structure, are turning over
independently.

However, before accepting this conclusion, it seems
necessary to examine if all of these enzymes are actually present in the same membrane. The membrane of
encoplasmic reticulum in liver cells may be quite
heterogeneous in composition and function. The electron-transport enzymes and the hydrolytic enzymes may
be located on different parts of the endoplasmic
reticulum, each group of enzymes forming a specialized
domain in the membrane. Moreover, since the enzymes
listed in Table II occupy only a small portion in the
total membrane protein of microsomes, their turnover
behavior may not represent the bulk membrane proteins
if they are not uniformly distributed over the whole
membrane.

Studies on the distribution of various enzymes in
microsomal membranes have already been carried out in
a few laboratories by sub-fractionating isolated microsomes (13-16). We have also studied this problem by
an immunochemical method using rabbit antibodies prepared against purified enzymes of rat liver microsomes

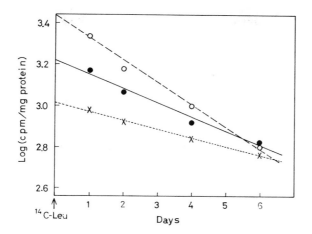

Figure 1: Turnover of Microsomal Enzymes in Rat
Liver. Open circles, NADPH-cytochrome c reductase.
Closed circles, Cytochrome b_5. X-signs, NADH-
cytochrome b_5 reductase.

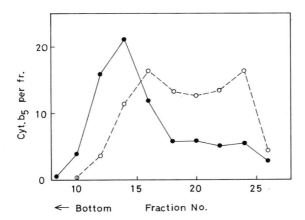

Figure 2: Sedimentation of Rat Liver Microsomes by
Anti-cytochrome b_5 Rabbit Immunoglobulin. Open
circles, Sedimentation pattern in the presence of
control immunoglobulin. Closed circles, Sedimentation pattern in the presence of anti-cytochrome
b_5 immunoglobulin.

327

(17). When added to the suspension of rat liver microsomes, the antibodies caused sedimentation of microsomal particles, and we could subfractionate the microsomes by centrifugation in a suitable concentration gradient of sucrose in the presence of the antibodies. Control immunoglobulin did not affect the sedimentation property of microsomes. Figure 2 shows an example of such experiments, in which microsomes were fractionated in the presence and absence of anti–cytochrome b_5 immunoglobulin, and the distribution of cytochrome b_5 among the subfractions was measured. Smooth microsomes with average vesicle diameter of 200 nm were used. The sedimentation of cytochrome b_5–containing microsomal vesicles by the antibody is seen from the Figure. The distribution of other microsomal enzymes as well as the distribution of total membrane protein and phospholipid were also studied. All of them showed a very similar shift in distribution pattern as shown in Fig. 2 for cytochrome b_5 when the antibody was added to the suspension of microsomes (data not shown). These results indicate that most microsomal vesicles contained cytochrome b_5, and that other microsomal enzymes were also almost uniformly distributed among the vesicles. Similar results were obtained when an antibody to NADPH-cytochrome $\underline{c}$ reductase was used.

These results indicate that the membrane of endoplasmic reticulum is not grossly heterogeneous in the distribution of enzymes although the microheterogeneity of the membrane has been suggested by the experiments with much smaller microsomal vesicles (12,13,15, 16). We are able to conclude that various kinds of microsomal enzymes in the same membrane turnover independently. The endoplasmic reticulum membrane in the liver cell does not seem to be degraded as a whole.

Secondly, I should like to discuss the stabilization or prevention of turnover of some particular microsomal enzymes when a drug, phenobarbital, is given to rats. As has been established about ten years ago, the administration of certain kinds of drugs including phenobarbital greatly increases the components of the NADPH-linked electron transport chain in liver microsomes, NADPH-cytochrome c reductase and cytochrome P-450, without affecting the activity of the NADH-linked electron transport chain. We studied the mechanism of this selective increase of NADPH-cytochrome c reductase in phenobarbital-treated rats, and we concluded that the stabilization of the enzyme is involved (18). We used guanidino-^{14}C-L-arginine to label the liver proteins to minimize the re-utilization of the labeled amino acid, and we observed almost complete cessation of degradation of NADPH-cytochrome c reductase when the animals were given phenobarbital.

Increased synthesis of the enzyme was also noticed with the drug-treated animals (18), but the drug-induced alteration in the turnover of NADPH-cytochrome c reductase was undoubtedly contributing to the observed increase of this specific enzyme in liver microsomes. Although the stabilization by the drug was also noticed for cytochrome b_5, all microsomal membrane proteins were not stabilized by phenobarbital administration to the animals. The turnover of total microsomal protein was only partially slowed by the drug (18).

We later observed another peculiar stabilizing effect of phenobarbital on the same reductase in the liver microsomes of drug-treated rats (19). When the early stage of incorporation of radioactive amino acids into microsomal enzymes was examined, a rapid initial loss of a significant amount of newly synthesized NADPH-cytochrome c reductase from microsomes was noticed, and this marked initial loss of the newly formed enzyme was almost completely prevented by a prior administration of phenobarbital to the animals. Figure 3 illustrates the result of an experiment on this subject.

The radioactive amino acid was injected into rats at time 0. The time course of incorporation of radioactivity into the reductase purified from isolated microsomes indicates that more than half of the newly synthesized reductase molecules do not become stable

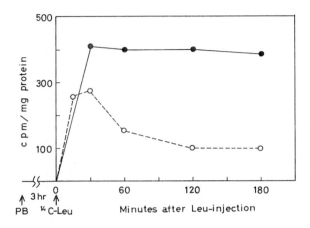

Figure 3:   Incorporation of ^{14}C–L–leucine into NADPH–
cytochrome <u>c</u> Reductase of Liver Microsomes. Open
circles, Control Rats without phenobarbital (PB)
injection. Closed circles, PB–treated rats.

membrane constituents (Fig. 3). They once appeared
in isolated microsomes, but were rather rapidly lost
from microsomes. Only less than half the newly synthesized reductase became the stable membrane component with a half-life of 70 hours. However, when
phenobarbital was given to the animals at 3 hours in
advance of the labeling with the radioactive amino
acid, there was no loss of radioactive newly synthesized reductase from microsomes during the initial
period of a few hours. This stabilizing effect of
phenobarbital in the early stage of membrane protein
formation may also be contributing to the increase of
this particular enzyme by the drug. This marked effect of the drug was not commonly observed for other
microsomal membrane enzymes, however. In the case of
cytochrome b_5, such initial rapid loss of newly synthesized enzyme from microsomes was not noticed even
without phenobarbital administration.

Thus, the turnover of the microsomal membrane proteins seems to be regulated at two steps. One is the
rapid turnover of the newly synthesized proteins before their incorporation into the membrane as integral
membrane constituents, and another is the slower turnover of the membrane-bound proteins with their characteristic half-lives. Drugs and other environmental
factors are able to affect the turnover of various
membrane proteins at either or both of these two steps
resulting in the decrease or increase of the total
amount of membrane or the contents of some specific
enzymes in the membrane.

I should like to mention one more interesting aspect of turnover studies on membrane proteins. It
has already been established that the different enzyme
proteins of the same membrane turnover independently
with their own characteristic half-lives. It would be
interesting to study next a different case where the
same enzyme protein is present in two different kinds
of membranes in the same cell. If the rate of turnover of an enzyme protein is affected by the properties of the membrane to which it is bound, the turnover of an enzyme present in a specific subcellular

organelle can be different from the same enzyme attached to another different organelle. The various kinds of membranes in the liver cell are quite different in their enzyme compositions and functions, but the presence of common enzyme components among them has been noticed.

NADH–cytochrome b_5 reductase and cytochrome b_5 are again promising candidates for the study on this subject because these two enzymes seem to be present not only in microsomes but also in a few other membranes in the liver cell; mitochondrial outer membrane (20) etc. A preliminary immunochemical investigation (21) suggested the similarity of the NADH–cytochrome b_5 reductase of mitochondrial outer membrane with its microsomal counterpart. More detailed recent studies in our laboratory (22) confirmed the identity of the reductases in these two membranes. Moreover, they are both located on the cytoplasmic side of the organelles exposed to the cytoplasm in the cell. Although the difference between microsomal cytochrome b_5 and the b–type cytochrome in mitochondrial outer membrane has recently emphasized (23), these two cytochromes have very similar properties in common (24). Both of them are also located on the cytoplasmic side of the membranes.

Turnover study on these two redox components of microsomes and mitochondrial outer membrane may tell us something about the specific character of membrane bound enzymes in their turnover. If there is any contribution of the membrane structure to the stability of enzyme protein in the cells, it will give us a clue to elucidate the mechanism of degradation of membrane protein constituents.

References

1. Omura, T., Siekevitz, P. & Palade, G. E.   J. Biol. Chem. 242, 2389 (1967).
2. Arias, I. M., Doyle, D. & Schimke, R. T.   J. Biol. Chem. 244, 3303 (1969).

3. Dehlinger, P. J. & Schimke, R. T. J. Biol. Chem. 246, 2574 (1971).
4. Takesue, S. & Omura, T. J. Biochem. 67, 259 (1970).
5. Ito, A. & Sato, R. J. Biol. Chem. 243, 4922 (1968).
6. Ito, A. & Sato, R. J. Cell Biol. 40, 179 (1969).
7. Akao, T. & Omura, T. J. Biochem. 72, 1245 (1972).
8. Kuriyama, Y. J. Biol. Chem. 247, 2979 (1972).
9. Okada, Y. & Omura, T. in preparation.
10. Akao, T. & Omura, T. J. Biochem. 72, 1257 (1972).
11. Edwards, P. A. & Gould, R. G. J. Biol. Chem. 247, 1520 (1972).
12. Bock, K. W., Siekevitz, P. & Palade, G. E. J. Biol. Chem. 246, 188 (1971).
13. Dallner, G., Bergstrand, A. & Nilsson, R. J. Cell Biol. 38, 257 (1968).
14. Glaumann, H. & Dallner, G. J. Cell Biol. 47, 34 (1970).
15. Schulze, H. U. & Staudinger, H. J. Z. physiol. Chem. 352, 1659 (1971).
16. Schulze, H. U., Ponnighaus, J. M. & Staudinger, H. J. Z. physiol. Chem. 353, 1195 (1972).
17. Kawajiri, K., Ito, A. & Omura, T., in preparation.
18. Kuriyama, T., Omura, T., Siekevitz, P. & Palade, G. E. J. Biol. Chem. 244, 2017 (1969).
19. Negishi, M. & Omura, T. J. Biochem. 72, 1407 (1972).
20. Sottocasa, G. L., Kuylenstierna, B., Ernster, L. & Bergstrand, A. J. Cell Biol. 32, 415 (1967).
21. Takesue, S. & Omura, T. Biochem. Biophys. Res. Commun. 40, 396 (1970).
22. Kuwahara, S., Okada, Y. & Omura, T., in preparation.
23. Fukushima, K. & Sato, R. J. Biochem. 74, 161 (1973).
24. Ito, A., in preparation.

BLOOD PRESSURE REGULATION BY PROTEINASE
AND ACTIVE PEPTIDES

Tatsuo Kokubu, Einosuke Ueda,and Kazutaka Nishimura

The Third Department of Medicine
Osaka University Medical School
Fukushima-ku, Osaka, Japan

Regulation by proteolytic enzymes acting on protein substrates in the blood stream is the subject of this paper. For instance, there are several active polypeptide forming systems such as the renin-angiotensin system and the kallikrein-kinin system. It is characteristic that active intermediate polypeptides, such as angiotensin and bradykinin which control the blood pressure, are produced by limited proteolysis.

On the other hand, there is other evidence that lung plays an important role in the production, release, and metabolism of vasoactive substances including antiotensin and bradykinin. It is widely accepted that the conversion of angiotensin I (inactive form) to angiotensin II (active form) as shown in Fig. 1 and the inactivation of bradykinin occur in the pulmonary circulation.

The present report contains biochemical and physiological studies of the angiotensin I converting enzyme and kininase in plasma and lung tissue, and also of the metabolic action of the lung on various vasoactive substances. In addition, we discuss the roles of the intermediate polypeptides produced by limited hydrolysis and of the pulmonary circulation in regulating the systemic blood pressure.

We have purified the angiotensin I converting enzyme from rabbit plasma. The enzyme activity was estimated by our bioassay method reported previously

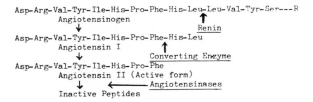

Figure 1:   Renin Angiotensin System.

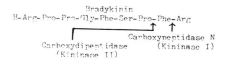

Figure 2:   Kininase I and II.

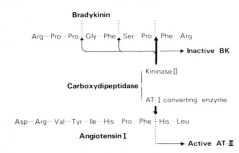

Figure 3:   Cleavage of Angiotensin I and Bradykinin by Carboxydipeptidase.

TABLE I.

Purification of Converting Enzyme

Steps	Total activity	Specific activity	Recovery	Fold
	(ng/h)	(ng/mg/h)		
Plasma	1479600	137	100.0	1.0
(NH₄)₂SO₄ Fractionation	525245	349	35.4	2.6
DEAE Sephadex A-50	163440	908	11.0	6.6
Sephadex G-200	138147	8570	9.3	63.0

(1). The activity of the enzyme was expressed in ng/mg/h. 200 ml of rabbit plasma was fractionated with ammonium sulfate from 1.6M to 2.2M saturation, followed by chromatography and gel filtration on a DEAE Sephadex A-50 column and Sephadex G-200 respectively. The final product had a specific activity of 8570 ng/mg/h showing a 63-fold purification from the original plasma (Table I). Five mg of angiotensin I was incubated with 290 μg of enzyme material at 37°C for 20 hrs. The incubation products were separated by means of high voltage paper electrophoresis. Five ninhydrin positive spots resulted. Using the amino acid autoanalyzer, these spots indicated Leu, angiotensin II, angiotensin I, His-Leu and His respectively. This result suggested that the enzyme had dipeptidase activity as well as converting enzyme activity. The enzyme preparation released His-Leu from the C-terminal of angiotensin I, hydrolyzed His-Leu, Leu-Gly and Leu-Gly-Gly, thereby suggesting the existence of a di- and a tri-peptidase activity. Furthermore, the enzyme preparation also inactivated bradykinin. These findings suggest that the converting enzyme might have the bradykinase activity at the same time. The enzyme did not hydrolyze angiotensin II.

We next attempted to separate the converting enzyme from the kininase by means of chromatography on DE-32, Bio-Gel A-15 and by electrophoresis, all without success. Next, as a possible method to differentiate these two enzyme activities, the bradykinin potentiating peptide B (BPPB), which had been known to have the specific inhibitory activity of kininase, and EDTA were examined. BPPB at a concentration of 10^5 pM caused a complete inhibition of converting enzyme activity and 80% inhibition of kininase activity. Both enzyme activities were inhibited by 10^{-3}M EDTA. Thus on the basis of effects of BPPB and EDTA, no difference between converting enzyme and kininase activity of our preparation could be demonstrated (2,3)

As to bradykinin inactivating enzymes, so-called kininase, two kinds of kininases have been reported. These are kininase I and kininase II as shown in Fig.

2. It has been assumed that the converting enzyme might be the same as kininase II releasing dipeptide from the C-terminal of bradykinin. Recently it was revealed that kininase II acted mainly in the pulmonary circulation. We therefore purified the converting enzyme from rabbit lung tissue and confirmed that it also had kininase activity at the same time. The converting enzyme and the kininase in plasma and in the tissue were compared using DEAE–Sephadex A–50 column chromatography and horizontal starch block electrophoresis. The converting enzyme in plasma and in the lung tissue were eluted at the same molarity of sodium chloride in linear gradient elution on DEAE Sephadex A–50. The two activities also migrated the same on starch block electrophoresis. Kininase activity always appeared with converting enzyme activity. We studied reaction products from angiotensin I after incubation with the converting enzyme preparation from lung tissue, using thin layer chromatography. Five products (Leu, His–Leu, angiotensin I, angiotensin II, and His) were observed. We conclude that the converting enzyme in lung tissue also might be the same as kininase II, so-called carboxydipeptidase.

Figure 3 shows the metabolic scheme of angiotensin I and bradykinin degradation by carboxydipeptidase, which has the converting enzyme activity and kininase II activity, in lung tissue. It is proposed that the carboxydipeptidase acts in the renin–angiotensin system and also in the kallikrein–kinin system, and thereby activates angiotensin I to pressor polypeptide, i.e. angiotensin II in plasma, and inactivating depressor peptide, bradykinin, in the lung. From these results I would like to emphasize that these two proteases might be identical and belong to a class of carboxydipeptidase. In the case of bradykinin as a substrate, dipeptides are released in order from the C-terminal. In the case of angiotensin I, however, the subsequent hydrolysis of the peptide does not occur after the release of dipeptide, His–Leu, from the C-terminal, perhaps because Pro is located in the second position from the C-terminal of angiotensin II. Thus when the substrate structures are different, the same enzyme shows a different mode of hydrolysis.

We suspect that the lung is metabolically active toward vasoactive substances, including angiotensin I and II and bradykinin. Thus, our interest was focused upon the metabolic action of the lung on various kinds of vasoactive substances. In order to study the metabolic action of the lung, we carried out in vivo experiments and perfusion experiments of rabbit heart-lung preparation (4). Rabbits were anesthetized with intravenous injections of pentobarbital sodium. A cannula was inserted into the aorta through the femoral artery and then fixed so that the top of the cannula was in the thoracic artery just above the diaphragm. Another cannula was fixed in the auricular vein, and the systemic blood pressure was recorded in the carotid artery with the help of a polygraph. Vasoactive substances were injected through the aortic cannula or auricular cannula and the responses of the systemic blood pressure were measured after each injection. The difference in the responses of the systemic blood pressure between these two routes for the same vasoactive substances was assumed to be the inactivation of the vasoactive substance in the pulmonary circulation. This assumption was based on the fact that the vasoactive substance, when injected through the auricular vein, affected the systemic blood pressure after passing through the lung. On the other hand, when injected through the aorta, it affected the systemic blood pressure directly without passing through the lung. Figure 4 shows that the systemic blood pressure response of vasoactive substance injected into the pulmonary circulation, when expressed as the percentage of the blood pressure response of the same dose of the vasoactive substance injected directly into the aorta in a normal rabbit. The amounts of the injected vasoactive substances were indicated in Fig. 4. The lower the percentage of the blood pressure response, the higher was the inactivation activity in the pulmonary circulation. The pressor effects of angiotensin I, angiotensin II, vasopressin, norepinephrine and epinephrine were not

339

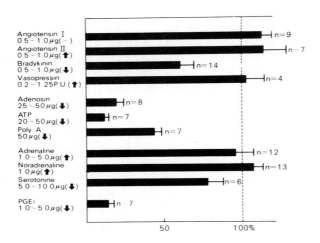

Figure 4: Response of Systemic Blood Pressure
    when Vasoactive Substances are Injected into
    Aorta and Auricular Vein in Normal Rabbit.

$$\frac{\text{BP response when injected through auricular vein (mmHg)}}{\text{BP response when injected through aorta (mmHg)}} \times 100 = \%$$

$\pm$S.E.   ($\uparrow\downarrow\sim$): Effect on blood pressure.

changed in the pulmonary circulation, but the depressor effects of bradykinin, serotonine, adenosine, ATP, poly A and prostaglandin E markedly decreased or were completely abolished by pulmonary circulation.

In the single perfusion experiments using the heart-lung preparation according to Vane (5), about 70 to 80% of angiotensin I was converted to angiotensin II after passing the pulmonary circulation once. There was a 100% recovery of perfused angiotensin II after a single passage through the pulmonary circulation. About 80 to 100% of bradykinin and prostaglandin E was inactivated after passing once through the apparatus. From the experimental results, it appears that the pressor substances, including angiotensin, vasopressin, epinephrine and norepinephrine, passed through the lung without change in pressor activity, whereas all the depressor substances were markedly affected.

We have also studied possible changes in the pulmonary metabolism of the vasoactive substances in the pathological lung. The experimental production of desquamative interstitial pneumonia-like lesions was made in rabbits according to the method of Moore et al. (6). The animals received intravenous injections of complete Freund's adjuvant at the dose of 0.5 mg with 7 days between the two injections. On the 3rd, 7th, 14th and 21st day of the treatment, the animals were used for the in vivo experiment. The massive cell accumulation in the alveolar spaces with marked cell infiltrations in the alveolar septa was observed microscopically in the lungs 3 days after the second injection. In rabbits 3 weeks after the second injection, the pulmonary lesions began to assume a granulomatous form with disappearing of cell accumulations in the alveolar spaces.

In order to compare the fate of vasoactive substances in the lung of normal rabbits and rabbits with the experimental pneumonitis, the equipotential dose of the vasoactive substance given via the auricular vein and the aorta was determined by comparing the systemic blood pressure response. The dose of angiotensin I, angiotensin II, bradykinin and prostaglandin E injected into the aorta, was 0.5 μg each, and the

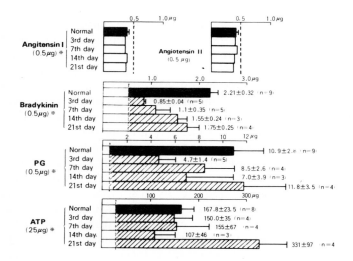

Figure 5: Equipotential Dose of Vasoactive Substance when Injected into Auricular Vein (Pulmonary Circulation) and Directly into Aorta in Rabbits with Experimental Pneumonitis.

* Doses of vasoactive substance directly into aorta.
** Equipotential doses, mean value ± S.E.

342

amount of ATP was 25 μg. As shown in Fig. 5 with
angiotensin I and II, no difference between the equipotential doses in normal rabbits and rabbits with
pneumonitis was observed through the experimental
period. However, the equipotential doses of bradykinin and prostaglandin given via the pulmonary circulation were significantly low on the 3rd day of the
treatment, then gradually increased, and they completely restored to the normal values on the 21st day
of the treatment. These results lead to the suggestion that the removal of the depressor substance in
the pulmonary circulation, especially bradykinin and
prostaglandin, might be disturbed in the pathological
lung, and much more depressor substances should escape
into the systemic circulation. These possible phenomenon might lead to a disease state such as hypotension. The systemic blood pressure levels of rabbits
with the experimental pneumonitis were lower than
those of normal rabbits, that is, the former was 83 ±
3.7 mmHg and the latter 113.5 ± 2.8 mmHg.

Next, the angiotensin I converting enzyme activity
of the rabbit lung extract was estimated according to
the method of Cushman et al. (7), a spectrophotometric
assay method measuring the rate of production of hip-
puric acid from hippryl–His–Leu. According to this
assay method, kininase II activity is also estimated.
The enzyme activity in normal rabbit lung extract was
3070 ± 510 μM/g/min, and in the pathological lung the
activity was 523 ± 94 μM/g/min on the 3rd day of the
treatment, 1302 ± 160 on the 7th day, 1445 ± 128 on
the 14th day and 2493 ± 280 on the 21st day. Carboxydipeptidase activity was significantly suppressed on
the 3rd day of the treatment, then gradually increased
and on the 21st day the activity was almost restored.

As to the inactivation of bradykinin in the lung,
the parallelism between the equipotential doses of
bradykinin in the in vivo experiment and the change
of the carboxydipeptidase activity of the lung tissue
was observed. But, in the case of angiotensin I,
there was no correlation between the results of the
in vivo experiment and the change of angiotensin I

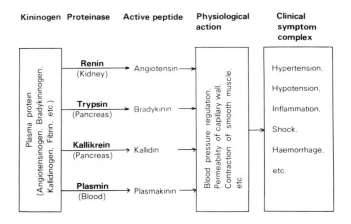

Figure 6: Metabolic Regulation by Proteolytic Enzymes.

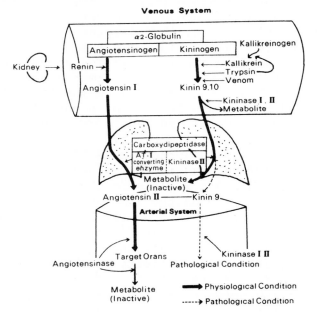

Figure 7: Metabolism of Vasoactive Peptides in Pulmonary Circulation.

converting enzyme activity in the lung tissue. We
plan to undertake further studies of the dissociation
of the reaction of the renin-angiotensin system and
the kallikrein-kinin system in the pathological condition.

Figure 6 lists several active polypeptide formation systems, including angiotensin, bradykinin, kal-
lidin and plasma kinin formation systems. The levels
of the resultant intermediate active peptides in blood
are controlled by various kinds of proteolytic enzymes
including renin, angiotensin I converting enzyme and
angiotensinases for angiotensin, and kallikrein and
kininase for bradykinin. The active peptides might
take part in a maintenance of homeostasis in the metabolic regulation. The failure of the process might
cause various clinical symptoms, such as hemorrhage,
inflammation, hypertension, hypotension and shock.

Figure 7 shows a scheme of metabolism of vasoactive
peptides in pulmonary circulation. Carboxydipeptidase,
which has the converting enzyme activity and kininase
II activity, acts in the renin-angiotensin system and
also in the kallikrein-kinin system, and thereby acti-
vating angiotensin I to pressor polypeptide (angiotensin II) and inactivating depressor polypeptide
(bradykinin) in the pulmonary circulation. This
brings angiotensin II into the systemic circulation
and distributes it to the vital organs. Hence, angiotensin II has the characteristics of a "circulating
hormone". On the other hand, in the physiological
condition, bradykinin, which was brought from the
venous blood into the pulmonary circulation, may be
almost completely inactivated in the pulmonary circulation by kininase except for pathological conditions,
such as carcinoid syndrome, inflammation of lung or
bronchogenic asthma. It is concluded that the pulmonary circulation might play an important role in the
regulation of the active peptide formation system and
in the systemic blood pressure regulation.

345

References

1. Ueda, E., Akutsu, H., Kokubu, T. & Yamamura, Y. Jap. Circulation J. 35, 801 (1971).
2. Ueda, E., Kokubu, T., Akutsu, H. & Yamamura, Y. Experientia 27, 1020 (1971).
3. Ueda, E., Kokubu, T., Akutsu, H. & Ito, T. Jap. Circulation J. 36, 583 (1972).
4. Ueda, E., Hatanaka, Y., Ito, T., Kokubu, T. & Yamamura, Y. Jap. Circulation J. 37, 1255 (1973).
5. Vane, J. R. Brit. J. Pharmacol. 12, 344 (1957).
6. Moore, R. D. & Schoenberg, M. D. Brit. J. Exp. Path. 45, 488 (1964).
7. Cushman, D. W. & Cheung, H. S. Biochem. Pharmacol. 20, 1637 (1971).

SUBJECT INDEX

A	5
B	6
C	7
D	8
E	9
F	0
G	1
H	2
I	3
J	4